# Classic Papers and Pioneers in Maxillofacial and Oral Surgery

Shahid R. Aziz • Michael D. Turner
Editors

# Classic Papers and Pioneers in Maxillofacial and Oral Surgery

Springer

*Editors*
Shahid R. Aziz
Division of Oral and Maxillofacial Surgery Department of Otolaryngology
Hackensack Meridian School of Medicine
Nutley, NJ, USA

Michael D. Turner
Division of Oral and Maxillofacial Surgery
Icahn School of Medicine at Mount Sinai
New York, NY, USA

ISBN 978-3-031-63245-7 ISBN 978-3-031-63246-4 (eBook)
https://doi.org/10.1007/978-3-031-63246-4



This Springer imprint is published by the registered company Springer Nature Switzerland AG
The registered company address is: Gewerbestrasse 11, 6330 Cham, Switzerland

*I would like to dedicate this work to my children (and co-authors) Aydin and Samina. My first and second heart sounds. There is no greater joy than being a father, and no prouder father than I. Also, deepest thanks to my parents, the late Dr. Mohammed Aziz and Dr. Fatima Aziz, themselves legends in their fields. I would also like to thank my co-editor Dr. Michael Turner for his efforts in helping this book come to fruition as well as all the contributors to this text. Special acknowledgement to my friend and colleague Dr. Joel Friedman who we lost prior to publication. Finally, to my Teresa: thank you for your unwavering kindness and support to my career.*

**—Shahid R. Aziz**

*This book is dedicated to my wife, Susie, and my children, Asher, Maya, and Alex. Thank you for your unwavering support and for giving me the time to read, write, and teach. Your love and patience have made this journey possible, and I am forever grateful. I am also deeply indebted to Daniel Buchbinder for his kindness, wisdom, guidance, and unwavering support, which have been instrumental in helping me achieve my professional goals. And finally, thank you to my co-editor Shahid Aziz for the decades of friendship and collaboration and for being a shining example of what it means to be a great human being.*

**—Michael D. Turner**

# Contents

# Introduction

# 1

Shahid R. Aziz and Michael D. Turner

Oral surgery (now more specifically oral and maxillofacial surgery) as we know is the surgical specialty of dentistry; it is also the field that provides a bridge between medicine and dentistry. Historically, its roots (no pun intended) lie as early as the Edwin Smith Papyrus (written 1501 BC). Interestingly, it is only last 175 years (which aligns with the evolution of general anesthesia in 1846) did the specialty truly evolve from exodontia to what it is today—a specialty dedicated to full scope care of the face: both hard and soft tissue.

In 2016, Roger Meyer succinctly listed some of the key milestones in the evolution of oral and maxillofacial surgery in the United States in his *Journal of Oral and Maxillofacial Surgery* letter to the editor: "Historical Milestones in Oral and Maxillofacial Surgery" [1]. These include:

1. World War I was the first time where modern facial skeletal and soft tissue trauma was encountered, forcing the dentist/surgeon to develop techniques still in use today.
2. The American Society of Exodontists (later, the American Society of Oral Surgeons and Exodontist, now American Association of Oral and Maxillofacial Surgeons) was established in 1918.
3. During World War II, based on World War I experience, oral surgeons became a key component of military surgical units for the care of war injuries to the face, mouth, and jaws.
4. The *Journal of Oral Surgery* (now the *Journal of Oral and Maxillofacial Surgery*) first published in 1943 and remains the official journal of the American Association.
5. Penicillin was introduced during World War II, a major breakthrough for treating life-threatening infections, particularly odontogenic.
6. The American Board of Oral Surgery was officially established in 1946, renamed the American Board of Oral and Maxillofacial Surgery in 1978.
7. Professor Hugo Obwegeser of the University of Zurich, in the mid-1960s, visited the United States and gave a series of seminal presentations on orthognathic surgery based on procedures he developed in the 1950s.
8. Combined MD and OMS programs were developed in the early 1970s and are now offered by more than half of all OMS residency programs in the United States.

S. R. Aziz (✉)
Division of Oral and Maxillofacial Surgery, Department of Otolaryngology, Hackensack Meridian School of Medicine, Nutley, NJ, USA
e-mail: azizsr@sdm.rutgers.edu; Shahid.aziz@hmhn.org

M. D. Turner
Division of Oral and Maxillofacial Surgery, Icahn School of Medicine at Mount Sinai, New York, NY, USA
e-mail: michael.turner@mountsinai.org



S. R. Aziz, M. D. Turner (eds.), *Classic Papers and Pioneers in Maxillofacial and Oral Surgery*, https://doi.org/10.1007/978-3-031-63246-4_1

9. In 1977, the name of the specialty association was updated to the American Association of Oral and Maxillofacial Surgeons, reflecting its evolving scope of practice.

This text, Classic Papers, evolved from an exploration by the editors of what we consider to be the landmark papers that contributed to the evolution of oral and maxillofacial surgery in the United States. Many of the chapters in this text reflect what is listed above. Beyond the paper, the editors were interested in who the author of said paper was, their legacy and contribution to our specialty. As such, we asked each chapter author to not just talk about the paper and its impact on today's oral and maxillofacial surgeon but also provide a biography of the person behind the classic paper.

The Great War (World War I) was a landmark period in the evolution of maxillofacial surgery. As such, the editors decided to separate this text into sections—pre-Great War, Great War, and post-Great War. We would like to thank all our contributors and hope that our readers will find this to be an enjoyable read and ultimately a reference for future maxillofacial surgeons.

## Reference

1. Meyer RA. Historical milestones in oral and maxillofacial surgery. J Oral Maxillofac Surg. 2016;74:2336–7.

# Part I

# Nineteenth Century Papers

# Case of Elongation of the Under Jaw and Distortion of the Face and Neck. The American Journal of Dental Science. Vol 9, No 2. January 1849

2

Shahid R. Aziz and Aydin M. Aziz

**Abstract**

Orthognathic surgery is considered to be one of the foundations of maxillofacial surgery. It is an area unique to the maxillofacial surgeon. Its early evolution is often credited to Vilray Blair, MD, the famed St. Louis plastic surgeon who, in conjunction with Edward Angle, developed organized orthognathic surgery. The most significant developments in twentieth century orthognathic surgery were based in Switzerland, Austria, and Germany, specifically involving Wassermund, Trauner, and Obwegeser, to name a few. What is often overlooked is the true origin of orthognathic surgery: Wheeling, Virginia, in 1847 (now Wheeling, West Virginia), by the surgeon Simon P. Hullihen, MD, DDS. Hullihen performed the first documented case of an osteotomy on the mandible to treat a malocclusion. While this was a post-traumatic surgery, this paper is considered to be the original written work describing what is now known as orthognathic surgery.

**Keywords**

Orthognathic surgery · Mandibular osteotomy · Simon Hullihen · Maxillofacial surgery · Wheeling · West Virginia · Father of Oral Surgery

S. R. Aziz (✉)
Division of Oral and Maxillofacial Surgery, Department of Otolaryngology, Hackensack Meridian School of Medicine, Nutley, NJ, USA
e-mail: azizsr@sdm.rutgers.edu; Shahid.aziz@hmhn.org

A. M. Aziz
School of Arts and Sciences, Class of 2027, University of Pennsylvania, Philadelphia, PA, USA
e-mail: ayaziz@sas.upenn.edu

Orthognathic surgery has evolved into one of the standards of care in oral and maxillofacial surgery. It is an area unique to the maxillofacial surgeon. What is often overlooked is the true origin of orthognathic surgery: a mandibular osteotomy performed by the surgeon Simon P. Hullihen, MD, DDS, in Wheeling West Virginia (Fig. 2.1). Hullihen wrote the first documented paper on the correction of skeletal malocclusion: "Case of Elongation of the Under Jaw and Distortion of the Face and Neck. The American Journal of Dental Science. Vol 9, No 2. January 1849." Hullihen wrote about a young woman severely burned as a child with a scar contracture causing a significant prognathism:

> Miss Mary S, aged 20, daughter of the Hon. Wm S., of Ohio, came to Wheeling in the Spring of 1848, to obtain relief from the effects of a very severe burn, which she received 15 years before. The burn was primarily confined to the neck and lower part of the face, and its cicatrix produced a



S. R. Aziz, M. D. Turner (eds.), *Classic Papers and Pioneers in Maxillofacial and Oral Surgery*,
https://doi.org/10.1007/978-3-031-63246-4_2

deformity of the most dreadful character. Her head was drawn forward and downward—the chin was confined within an inch of the sternum—the under-lip was so pulled down that the mucous membrane of the left side came far below the chin—the under jaw was bowed slightly downward, and elongated, particularly in its upper portion, which made it project about 1 in. and three eighths beyond the upper jaw. She was barely able to turn her head to either side. She could not close her jaws but for an instant, and then only by bowing her head forward; she could not retain her saliva for a single instant, and as might be expected, her articulation was very indistinct (Fig. 2.2a, b).

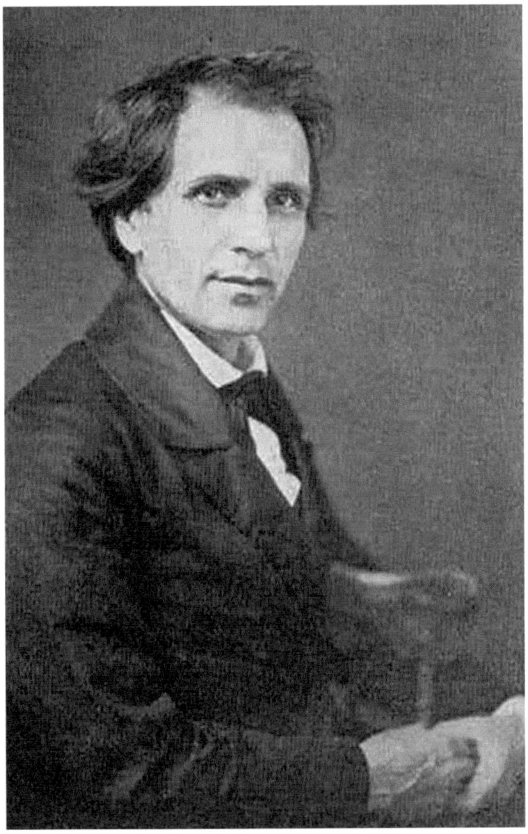

**Fig. 2.1** Simon P. Hullihen, MD, DDS (1810–1857)

Hullihen decided that a three-phase surgical plan was in order: the initial procedure focused on correcting the skeletal deformity of the mandible, followed by resection of the large cicatrix of the right face and neck and then correction of the lower lip defect. Hullihen noted that correcting the malocclusion was most important—it provided for the restoration of function. He noted that there were edentulous spaces between the first premolar and the canine on the right; in the left mandible, there was a space between the premolars. Most likely, these spaces were secondary to the cicatrix distracting anterior mandible as it developed. Hullihen used these spaces to treat the prognathism by performing wedge resection of bone bilaterally combined with what is now known as an anterior subapical osteotomy, as described by Kole in 1959 (Fig. 2.3).

The operation was commenced by sawing out, in a V shape, the elongated portions, together with the first bicuspid on the left side, each section extending about three-fourths of the way through the jaw. I then introduced a bistoury at the lower point of the space from which the section was re- moved on the right side, and pushed through the soft parts, close to and in front of the jaw, until it came out at the lower point of the space on the left side. The bistoury was then withdrawn, and a slender saw introduced in the same place, and the upper three fourths of the jaw, containing the six front teeth was sawed off on a horizontal line ending at the bottom of the spaces before named.

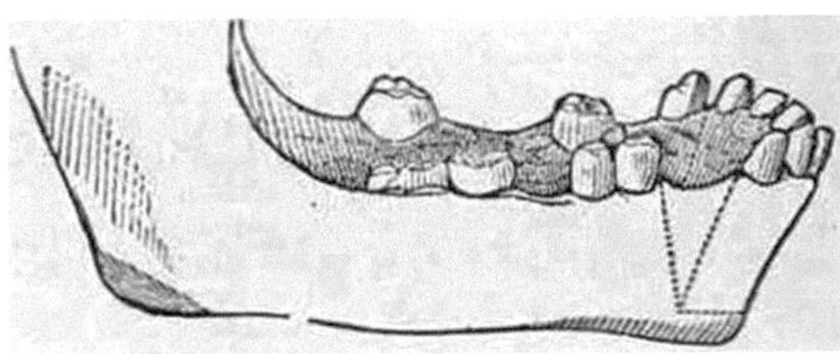

**Fig. 2.3** Preoperative mandible

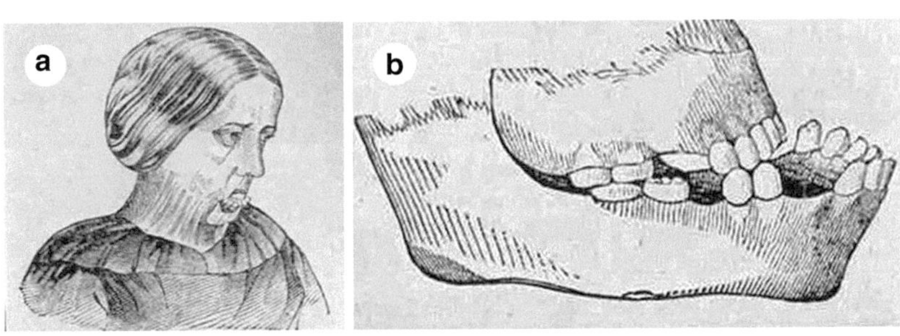


**Fig. 2.2** (**a**) Preoperative appearance. (**b**) Preoperative occlusion

Once the bone wedges were removed and the osteotomy completed, Hullihen then took an impression of the new mandibular occlusion, created a stone cast, and fabricated a silver plate (occlusal splint) combined with maxillomandibular fixation to immobilize the anterior mandible in its new position and facilitate bony healing. Postoperatively, Hullihen noted that the patient was relatively comfortable, without any significant complications. He left the splint on for 6 weeks to allow for bony union.

The second phase of surgery was performed on July 31, 1848. Hullihen excised the large cicatrix, which extended from the right cheek to the clavicle and sternum. This cicatrix prevented the patient from any significant movement of her head. He reconstructed the residual defect with a pedicled deltoid flap, sutured into place with "fine thread sutures." Hullihen dressed the flap with adhesive plaster. Unlike the prior operation, the patient's postoperative course at this point was a bit more involved. Hullihen wrote that she had what appears to be a psychotic episode postoperatively, perhaps from the analgesia given. The third and final surgery, performed 2–3 weeks after the second, was focused at correcting the lower lip deformity. "The underlip, from being dragged down and greatly stretched by the former projection of the under jaw, was rendered greatly too large—so much so that it pouted out an inch or more further than the upper lip." Hullihen decided to close this in a V-Y fashion (Fig. 2.4a, b).

In his article, Hullihen drew a rendering of the patient 3 weeks after the final surgery, illustrating a remarkable transformation: her prognathism was corrected and there was a restoration of facial/neck form (Fig. 2.5).

In light of this surgery taking place in a preantibiotic as well as preanesthetic era, what he accomplished is remarkable. Hullihen's lack of a modern dental education is, however, evident. While the prognathism was corrected, but the patient was left with an edge-to-edge occlusion anteriorly (Fig. 2.6). This could be from a combination of surgical limitations and/or resulted from a lack of formal dental/orthodontic training in occlusion. In addition, Hullihen performed this surgery 50 years before Edward Angle's classic treatise on the Classification of Occlusion. The cephalometric analysis used by today's orthognathic surgeon was developed 100 years after Hullihen's surgery. Hullihen also did not comment on the complications of this orthognathic

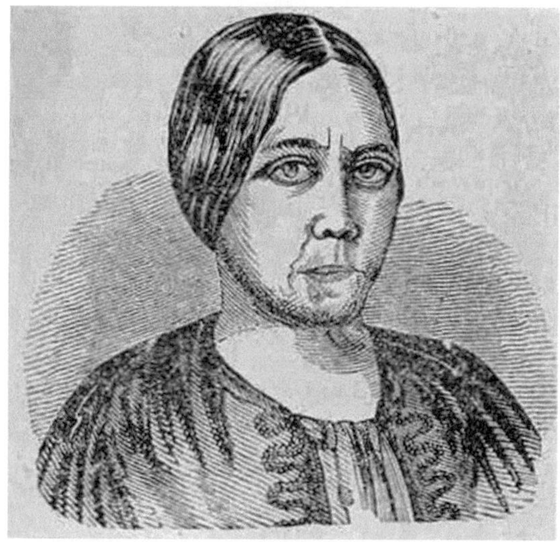

**Fig. 2.5** Postoperative appearance

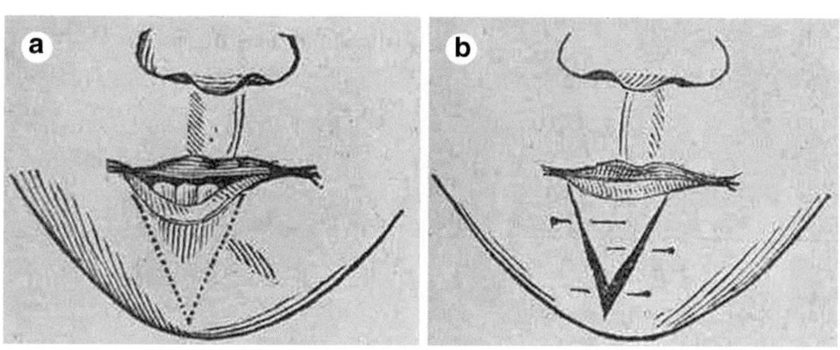

**Fig. 2.4** (**a**, **b**) V-Y closure of lip

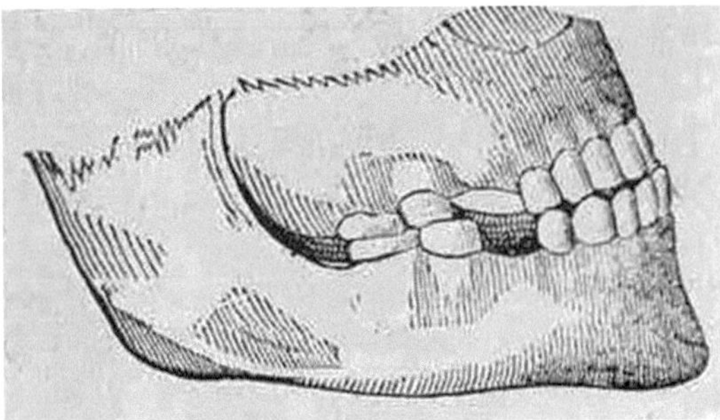

**Fig. 2.6** Postoperative occlusion

surgery. Mandibular subapical osteotomies place the mental foramen/neurovascular bundle at risk. In addition, preoperative radiographic evaluation must be used in treatment planning to avoid the mental neurovascular bundle as well as tooth root apices. Hullihen never documented the status of the mental nerves bilaterally, although it is likely that the nerve on the right, involved in the cicatrix, was damaged or non-existent after the burn injury. Without radiographs, Hullihen could only guess at the horizontal cut in the mandible to avoid the apices of the involved teeth. He did not make mention of tooth vitality postoperatively, as well.

Obviously the treatment planning for a case such as this would be significantly different by todays maxillofacial surgeon—osteotomies combined with potential microvascular reconstruction perhaps. Hullihen, however, given the technology of the nineteenth century, provided this young woman a great service.

Simon Hullihen was born in Western Pennsylvania on December 10, 1810, to a family of Irish farmers. He was the second of 3 boys. Hullihen's early childhood was uneventful until age 9, when he fell into a lime kiln, severely burning both legs. This injury left Hullihen bedridden for 2 years, under the constant care of local physicians. It was this experience that initiated his interest in medicine. Over the next several years, Hullihen spent time observing the local physicians, as well as working on his father's farm—it was a combination of the mechanical development and a taste for science that ultimately led him to develop a career in oral and maxillofacial surgery.

Hullihen went on to receive his medical degree from Washington Medical College in Baltimore in 1832 at the age of 22. He initially stayed on as an instructor, followed by brief practice in Canton, OH, and Pittsburgh, PA. It was his time in Pittsburgh when he met his wife-to-be, Elizabeth Fundenburg. They married in April 1835. Immediately following his marriage, Hullihen left via steamboat for Kentucky, where he planned to establish practice. He unfortunately became gravely ill and disembarked the boat in Wheeling, VA, to seek medical attention. After spending time in Wheeling, Hullihen decided that this was the place to settle. He announced his intention to devote his practice to dentistry and surgery of the head, neck, and oral cavity. The Wheeling medical community greeted his arrival with scorn; at the time, most dentists were of the "barber-surgeon" genre, rarely classically trained in medicine or dentistry. Other Wheeling physicians wondered why Hullihen, educated as a physician, would devote his career to dental surgery. Ultimately, he was met with significant mistrust. As a practical joke, a few months after Hullihen opened his practice, 2 medical students presented Hullihen with a chicken with a broken leg, requesting treatment. Rather than turn the "patient" away, allowing himself to be the victim of this joke, Hullihen accepted the chicken and subsequently splinted the leg, with the medical students as his surgical assistants. He then told these men "you must leave this patient with me for about ten days, during which time he should be kept under a barrel in my cellar and provided with proper diet. At the end of that time you will please call for him." After 2 weeks, the medical students did not return to collect their chicken. Undaunted, Hullihen returned the chicken to them with a fee of $20. Payment was subsequently refused; rather than leave the matter where it lay, Hullihen sought legal means, sued the students for his fee, and won.

Hullihen focused primarily on oral surgery. He developed a reputation for surgical excellence and catered to a patient base throughout the Ohio River Valley and beyond. Hullihen's meticulous records give a history of his surgical cases during the last 10 years of his life:

Cataract: 200 cases
Harelip: 100 cases
Cleft palate: 50 cases
Cancer (oral): 150 cases
Antrum: 200 cases
Strabismus: 100 cases
Making new nose: 25 cases
Making new lips: 50 cases
Making new underjaws: 10 cases
General surgery: 200 cases

He became particularly well known for his treatment of cleft lip and palate. Hullihen advocated surgical lip repair in infancy, before the eruption of dentition. He also used an "adhesive strap" from one cheek to another prior to surgery.

By thus confining the cheeks forward, a force is obtained and exerted upon the jaw, sufficiently great to close in a few weeks the widest cleft of the alveolar arch, and at the same time correct any projections of its process. As soon as the cleft edges of the alveolar arch are brought together so as to touch each other in the slightest manner, the operation for the cure of the harelip may be properly performed.

Perhaps what is most interesting is while it is now common to repair cleft lips in the first year of life, Hullihen did this before the advent of anesthesia! Hullihen noted that cleft palates required a significant amount of patient cooperation and therefore required surgery later in life. He advocated waiting until the child was 9 or 10 years of age. Hullihen also fabricated obturators for adult cleft palate patients.

For his leadership in oral surgery, the Baltimore College of Dentistry (now the University of Maryland Dental School) awarded Hullihen an honorary Doctorate of Dental Surgery in 1842. Although he had no formal dental training, Hullihen was a strong proponent of a sound medically based dental curriculum to elevate the profession from its barber-surgeon ancestry to the level of the medical profession. He later gave the Valedictory Address to the school's graduating class of 1850, in which he noted that dental education needed "to combine in the same person a thorough medical and mechanical education. An efficacious union of medical and mechanical skill is the only course, the only plan to make an accomplished Dental Surgeon."

Hullihen's most lasting legacy in Wheeling was founding Wheeling Hospital, in which the first hospital dental unit was created. Tragically, his brilliant career was suddenly cut short. On March 27, 1857, at the age of 47, Hullihen died of complications from typhoid pneumonia, contracted from exposure after being overheated in the operating theater at Wheeling Hospital. In his brief career of 22 years, Hullihen performed over 1100 maxillofacial surgeries. As word spread through Wheeling, the town declared his death a "public calamity." His obituary read, "amongst American surgeons he had no superior, probably no equal. In dentistry he was not equaled in America. With all these gifts of nature and attainment in science and art, a few hours' sickness brought him down to the gates of death."

To honor him, the Wheeling community erected a 30-foot marble monument in Wheeling's Mount Wood Cemetery, which still stands today. The exhaustive research of Hullihen's career by Edward Ambrecht, an oral surgeon in Wheeling, led to his being recognized as the "Father of Oral Surgery" in 1936. To commemorate this honor, the Wheeling Dental Society held Hullihen Day on August 18, 1936. The American Association of Oral and Maxillofacial Surgeons dedicated their 55th annual meeting to Hullihen's memory.

Simon Hullihen's contributions to our specialty were enormous. His work, coupled with that of James Garretson, Chalmers Lyons, Truman Brophy, and others, paved the way for organized oral and maxillofacial surgery and elevated the dental profession as a whole from a "trade" to a respectable, intellectual branch of medicine.

## Further Reading

Ambrecht EC. Hullihen, the oral surgeon. Int J Orthod Oral Surg. 1937;23(511, 598, 711):377.

Editors' Table. N Am Med Chir Rev. 1858;2:19.

Goldwyn R. Simon P. Hullihen. Plast Reconstr Surg. 1973;52:250.

Hullihen SP. Hare-lip and its treatment. Am J Dent Sci Ser 1. 1844;4:244.

Hullihen SP. Case of elongation of the underjaw and distortion of the face and neck, caused by a burn, successfully treated. Am J Dent Sci. 1849;9:157.

# 3 Dr. James Edmund Garretson, MD, DDS Surgical Education. The Dental Cosmos. Vol 18, pp186–188. November, 1866

Jessica S. Lee and Gregg A. Jacob

*I beg therefore to suggest to you that a period has now arrived when the conviction is forced upon us that this intelligence, as exhibited both in and out of the dental profession, demands and compels that, for the support of the doctorate assumed by the dentist, the greatest change must be effected in the matters of his education and duties; for his present scientific attainments and sphere of duties are too restricted.... This enlarged sphere consists in the conversion of the present specialty into that of Oral Surgery.*

*—James E. Garretson, MD, DDS. A communication read before the Association of the Colleges of Dentistry, at a meeting held in Philadelphia, Oct. 17, 1866. The Dental Cosmos. Vol 18, pp 186–188. November 1866.*

**Abstract**

The field of oral surgery, the first recognized specialty of dentistry, was developed and introduced by American surgeon James Edmund Garretson, MD, DDS, and created out of a necessity to bridge the gap between dentistry and medicine. By combining dental and surgical education, Garretson's vision was to equip his graduates with the knowledge and skill of oral surgeons: "the specialty to mean to the community the treatment of every disease of the mouth and associate parts, just as ophthalmic surgery means to the community the treatment of the hundred diseases of the eye, its cavity, and associate parts." Garretson's contributions to the field of oral surgery and his role as a pioneer in the creation of the specialty have helped forge a path for generations of surgeons to follow and expand the specialty of oral surgery.

**Keywords**

James Edmund Garretson · Oral surgery education · Oral surgery specialty · Surgical education

J. S. Lee (✉) · G. A. Jacob
Division of Oral and Maxillofacial Surgery, Department of Otolaryngology, Icahn School of Medicine at Mount Sinai, Mount Sinai Health System, New York, NY, USA

Northeast Facial and Oral Surgery Specialists, LLC, Florham Park, NJ, USA
e-mail: drlee@nefoss.com; drjacob@nefoss.com

The field of oral surgery, the first recognized specialty of dentistry, was developed and introduced by American surgeon James Edmund Garretson, MD, DDS (Fig. 3.1), and created out of a necessity to bridge the gap between dentistry and medicine. Garretson argued that dental trainees


S. R. Aziz, M. D. Turner (eds.), *Classic Papers and Pioneers in Maxillofacial and Oral Surgery*,
https://doi.org/10.1007/978-3-031-63246-4_3

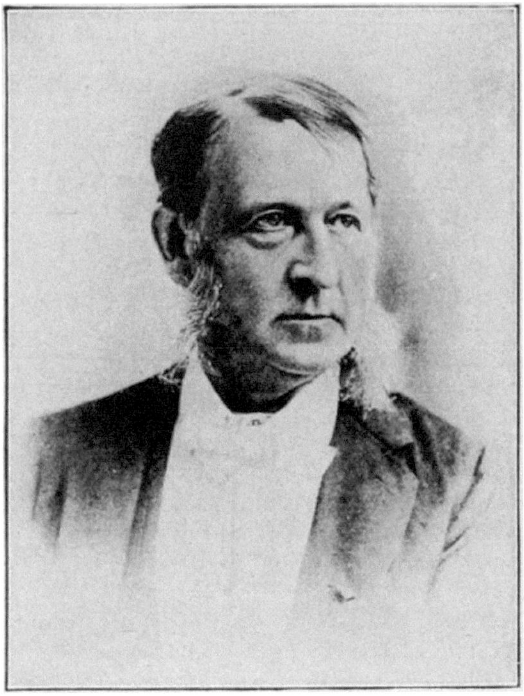

**Fig. 3.1** James Edmund Garretson, MD, DDS

graduated with an "inability to treat any disease outside of those associated with a few simple semi-vital organs, and which disease require for treatment much more the skill of a mechanician than that which the world recognizes as a doctor" [1].

Garretson was also concerned about the role of dentists in the medical community as "their attainments are understood by the community to be not of the same general character as that of other regular specialists, proven by the fact that, while all other specialists are understood as being proper doctors, and so received and consulted, the dentist is not" [1].

With an announcement to the Association of the Colleges of Dentistry on October 17, 1866, Garretson proposed a curriculum to train dental graduates in the study of general surgery.

> To this end, the student entering this school [Philadelphia Dental College] has offered to him every advantage in the way of the study of general surgery that is presented in any university or college in the country. Dissections, clinical observations, attention on didactic and demonstrative discourses, are necessary to his obtaining the highest honors of the school, or of receiving its indorsement as an oral surgeon, such general study being accepted as absolutely necessary to the position assumed [1].

Garretson stated that with this change in curriculum, graduates would be afforded a "wider field of work open to them" and their additional training would "stamp their entire equality with any and all medical practitioners." Further, he proposed that graduates of this new curriculum would be "surgeons by education, equal to any demand that emergencies may at any time make upon them, whether on the railway train, on the battle-field, or called hastily from the privacy of the office; yet presents its graduates as specialists" [1].

By combining dental and surgical education, Garretson's vision was to equip his graduates with the knowledge and skill of oral surgeons: "the specialty to mean to the community the treatment of every disease of the mouth and associate parts, just as ophthalmic surgery means to the community the treatment of the hundred diseases of the eye, its cavity, and associate parts" [1].

At the time of this announcement in 1866, Garretson himself did not have the title of oral surgeon at his institution until the first official recognition of oral surgery as a specialty was given in 1869, at which time Garretson was appointed Professor of Oral Surgery at the Hospital of the University of Pennsylvania. In the same year, Garretson published his work on *Diseases and Surgery of the Mouth and Jaws and Associated Parts* which was used as part of the curriculum by several dental colleges in existence at that time (Figs. 3.2 and 3.3) [2].

James Edmund Garretson was born on October 18, 1828, in Wilmington, Delaware. His studies in dentistry began with a Dr. Thatcher of Wilmington in 1850 and eventually began practicing in Woodbury, New Jersey. He entered as a student into the Philadelphia College of Dental Surgery in 1854 and received his dental degree in February 1856. Not completely satisfied with his doctorate degree in dentistry, Garretson matriculated into the University of Pennsylvania and earned his doc-

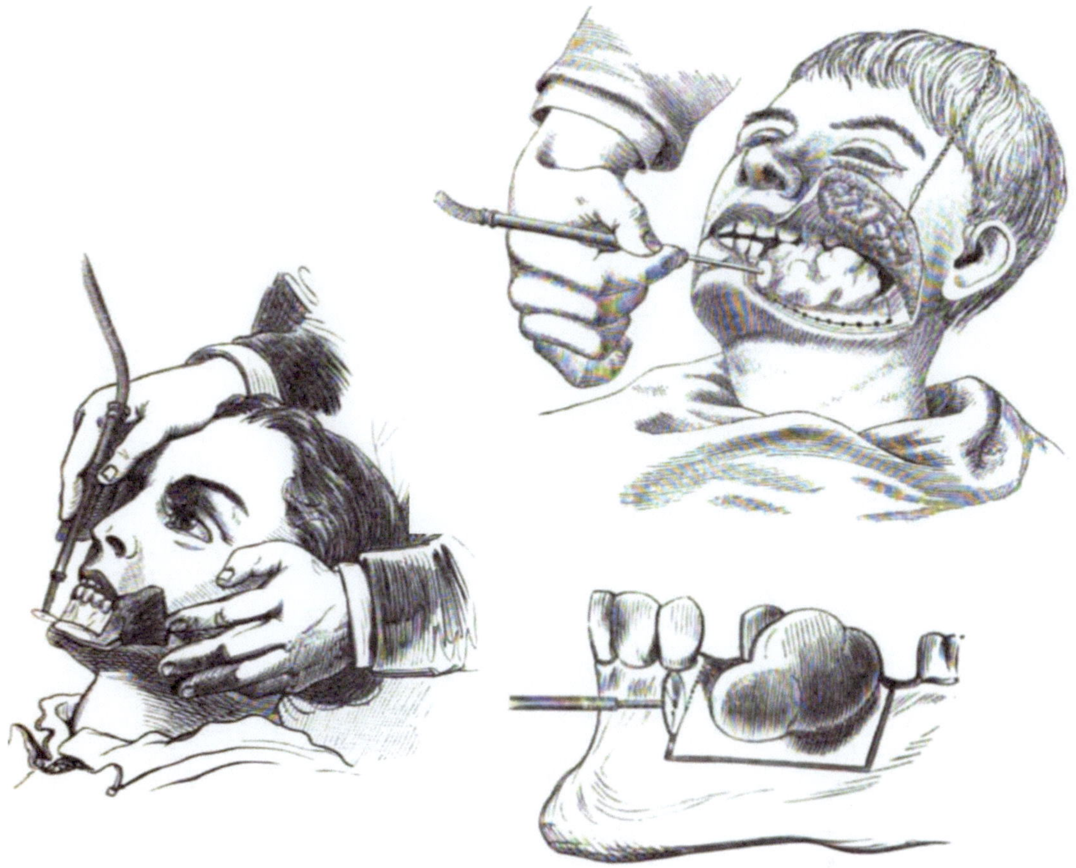

**Fig. 3.2** Garretson's illustrations of mandibular resection in the chapter "Exsections of the Maxillary Bones," in "A System of Oral Surgery," 4th Edition, J.B. Lippincott, Philadelphia, 1884

torate in medicine in 1859 and was married to Beulah Craft of Upper Greenwich, New Jersey, later that same year. Garretson had a deep passion for the study of anatomy and surgery and was appointed Director of the Philadelphia School of Anatomy in 1862, then entered the Philadelphia Dental College as Professor of Anatomy and Surgery shortly thereafter in 1864, during which time he offered his surgical services in military hospitals during the American Civil War (1861–1865) [3].

It was during his time at Philadelphia Dental College where Garretson seemingly began to develop and establish the specialty of oral surgery after which an official introduction of the specialty was announced by Garretson in 1866. Garretson was cognizant of the crudeness that characterized the surgical procedures of the head, face, and jaws and believed that the special training and many of the operative methods of the dentist were, with suitable modification, directly applicable to surgery within the specialty of oral surgery. Further, Garretson practiced within his new specialty with healthy conservatism and was aware of the importance of the cosmetic nature of his surgeries and, therefore, designed his incisions intraorally to avoid external incisions and scars as much as possible [3].

His conservatism also extended to the preservation of tissues of the oral cavity with his cardinal principle stating never to remove healthy tissue that might in any degree help to bring about a normal restoration of function within the territory of the procedure. Garretson's procedures on the mandible displayed this conservatism as well as it was his custom to leave a thin basilar rim of

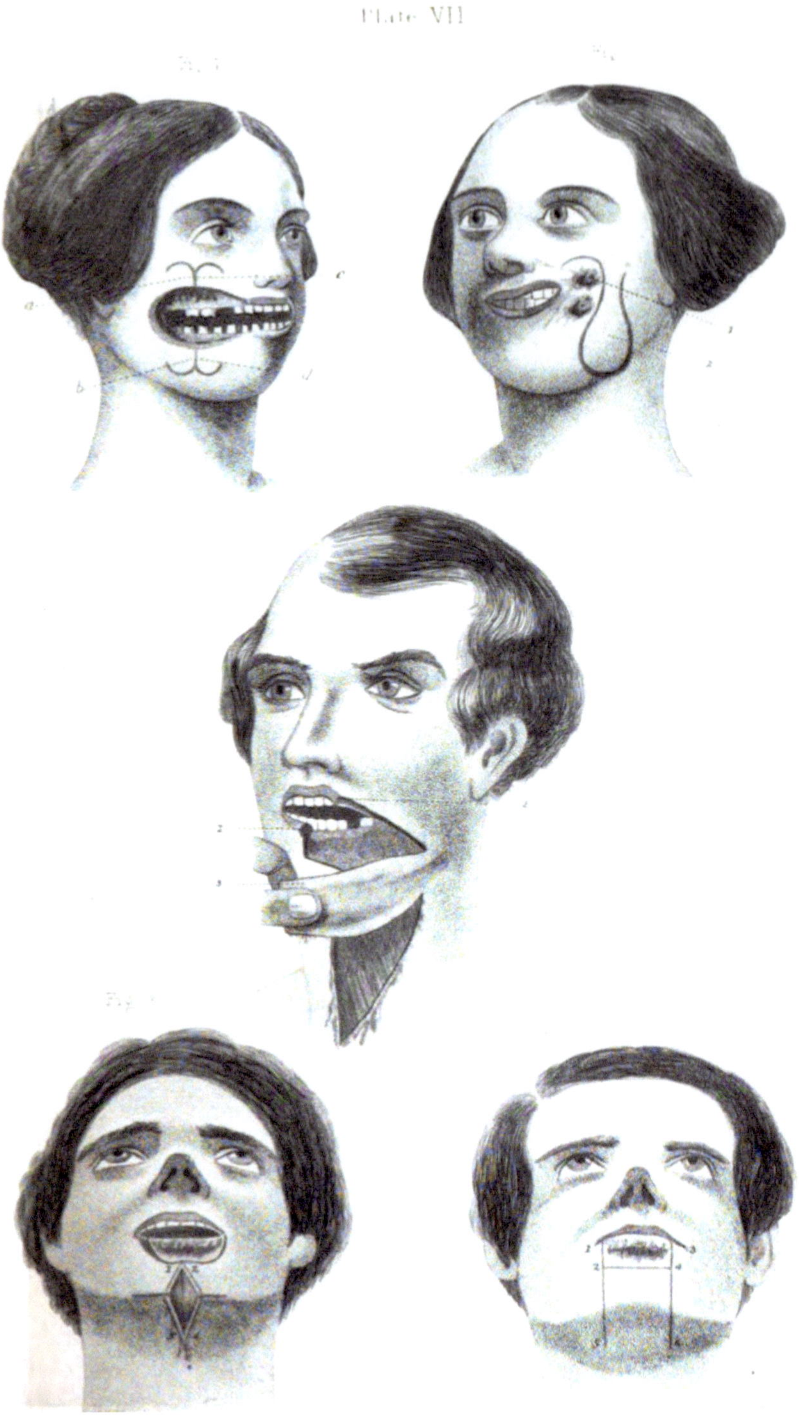

**Fig. 3.3** Garretson's illustrations of procedures of the cheek and lips in the chapter "Operations Upon the Lips and Cheek," in "A System of Oral Surgery," 4th Edition, J.B. Lippincott, Philadelphia, 1884

bone and periosteum to be used as a base for a denture. Garretson's success in his surgical procedures was also made possible by the use of the Bonwill dental engine (Fig. 3.4) and applied the use of this rotary instrument in bone surgery, namely the jaws but also the neurocranium [4].

In the early days of the development and adoption of the specialty of oral surgery, Garretson was criticized by his medical colleagues for the

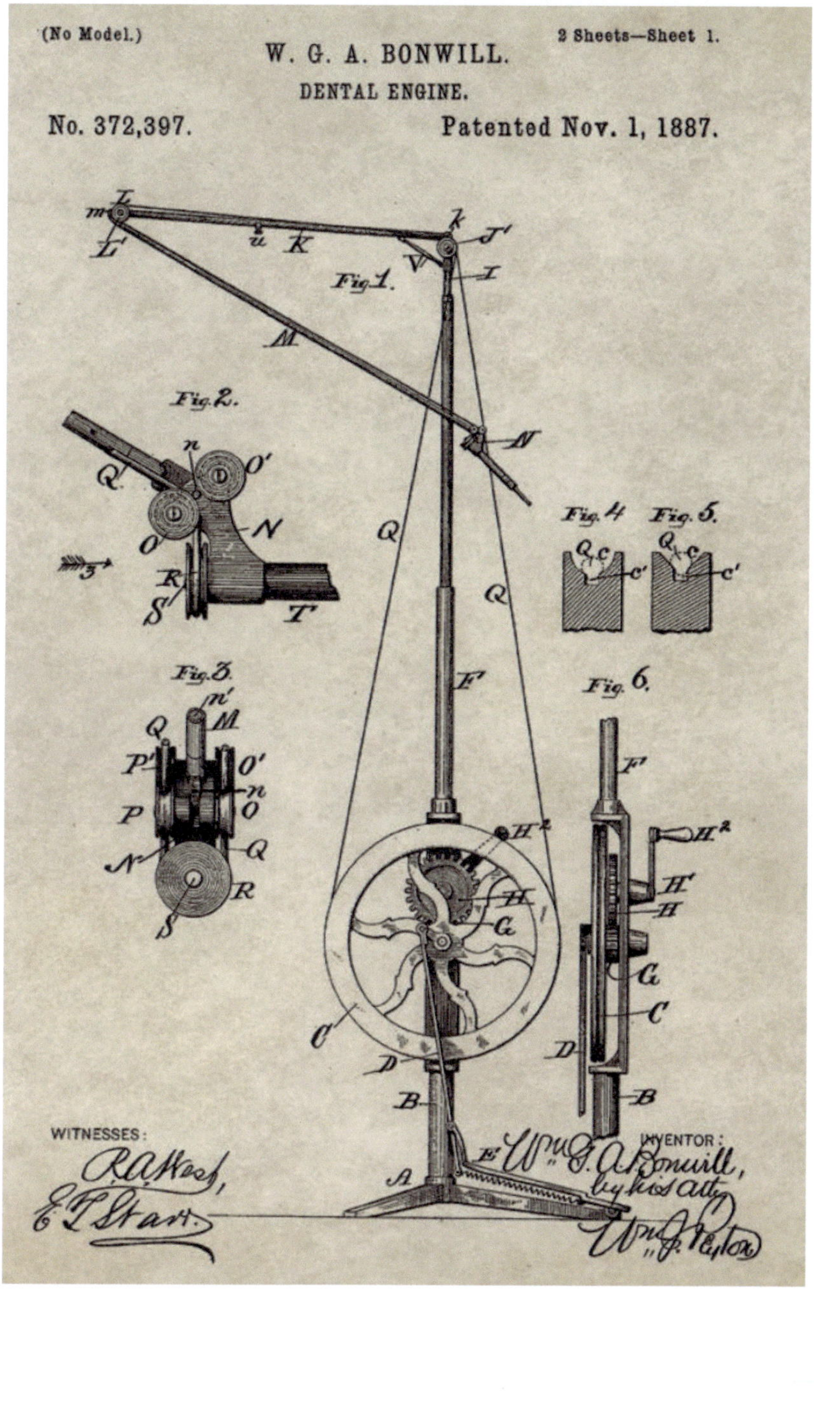


**Fig. 3.4** A sketch of Bonwill's dental engine utilized by Garretson

creation of the specialty as it was deemed "unnecessary" but the success of his surgical procedures was in strong contrast to the results obtained by the general surgeons who lacked the dental knowledge and skill possessed by Garretson.

Garretson was appointed Oral Surgeon to the Hospital of the University of Pennsylvania in 1869 but left in 1878 to return to the Philadelphia Dental College as Professor of Anatomy and Surgery and was subsequently appointed Dean of the Philadelphia Dental College in 1880 where he remained until his death in 1895 [3]. During Garretson's tenure at the Philadelphia Dental College, a formal curriculum outlining the training program for oral surgery was finalized.

> With the present session, the faculty of the Philadelphia Dental College inaugurates a change in the programme of the school which can scarcely fail in meeting with a hearty approval on the part of the profession at large, inasmuch as it offers opportunity for the most extensive surgical education, while at the same time the periods of progressive steps are left optional with the matriculates. The future of the specialty the faculty does not take it upon itself to decide; that great change, however, is not far off, cannot be overlooked nor denied. With a majority, the practice of the specialty is limited strictly to dentistry. By a constantly enlarging minority it is being extended to cover the ground of what is becoming more and more familiarly known as Oral Surgery. Members of the medical profession are constantly coming into the specialty and dental graduates aspire more and more to a general education in medicine. It is the object the change now made to complete a link so evidently uniting the two professions [4].

In place of the usual single course for dentistry, Garretson's new curriculum was now separated into three courses with separate examinations to demonstrate mastery of each course.

- *Course 1 - This is the regular dental course of the College; it extends over a period of two Winter sessions of five months each, with the Spring and Fall courses (four months) in addition. The degree conferred is Doctor of Dental Surgery.*
- *Course 2 - This course of five months is designed for the instruction of graduates of respectable Medical Colleges in dentistry proper. While the full curriculum of the School is open to the student of this course, he will be expected to pay special attention to the instruction of the Professors of Operative, Mechanical and Practice Dentistry.*
- *Course 3 - Arrangements have been made with the Jefferson Medical College, whereby students of the Philadelphia Dental College may obtain the two degrees, D.D.S. and M.D., in three years. Students taking this third course will be required during the second year to pursue extra studies in Surgery, practice of medicine and obstetrics* [4].

Due to the significant contributions made by the creation of this new specialty, the college became known as the Philadelphia Dental College and Hospital of Oral Surgery. With the growth of the specialty within the college, the need for appropriate facilities in which oral surgery could be practiced also increased. Initially, a small room was rented on the fourth floor of an adjoining building to the dental college with a door cut through for access, furnished with two cots, a few sheets, and a place to keep dressings. The food was obtained from a nearby restaurant and students served in the capacity of nurses [4].

As the demands of the hospital became greater, more rooms were procured to accommodate patients traveling from all parts of the United States and Canada. Garretson obtained rooms over the Third National Bank and was named the "Medico-Chirurgical Hospital." The Medico-Chirurgical Hospital (Fig. 3.5) was a facility that could accommodate the needs of the specialty of oral surgery, having male and female wards, two resident physicians always on duty, an apothecary, a matron, and a janitor together with a corps of trained nurses and attendants. It was with the creation of this facility that oral surgery was taught as regularly and as systematically as dentistry proper [4].

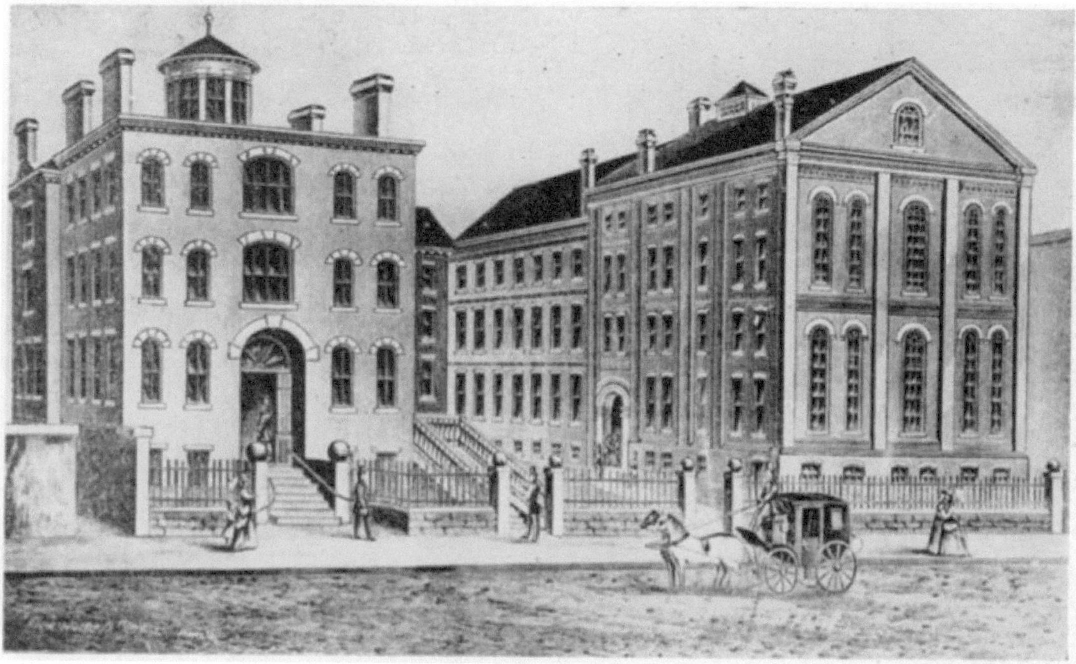

**Fig. 3.5** Medico-Chirurgical Hospital and College and Philadelphia Dental College. FAGGART, HAROLD L., and James E. Garretson. "DR. JAMES E. GARRETSON AND THE FIRST HOSPITAL OF ORAL SURGERY." Bulletin of the History of Medicine 17:4 (1945), Fig. 4 and Fig. 9. © 1945 Johns Hopkins University Press. (Reprinted with permission of Johns Hopkins University)

Garretson's surgical techniques and achievements throughout his career were documented in his textbook *System of Oral Surgery*, which was first published in 1868 with the sixth and last edition published in 1895. The last edition of the book demonstrated a culmination of Garretson's lifelong work and contribution to not only the establishment of oral surgery but also the continual evolution of the profession during his career. His earlier scientific publications included over 100 articles in the "Dental Cosmos," but Garretson was also a contributor to the general literature under the pen name of *John Darby* with publications including "Brushland," "Hours with John Darby," "Thinking and Thinkers," "Odd Hours of a Physician," "Nineteenth Century Sense," and "Man and His World" [5].

Garretson died on October 26, 1895, at his home in Lansdowne, Pennsylvania. To honor Garretson's creation of the specialty of oral surgery, on September 20, 1897, Philadelphia Dental College was renamed the Philadelphia Dental College and Garretson Hospital of Oral Surgery (Fig. 3.6), which later merged with and became known as Temple University in 1910 [4]. Garretson's contributions to the field of oral surgery, however, transcend a building or school and his role as a pioneer in the creation of the specialty has helped forge a path for generations of surgeons to follow and expand the specialty of oral surgery.

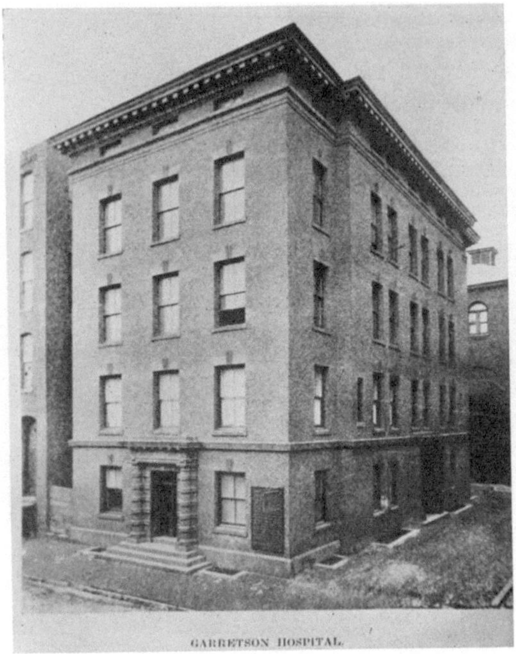


**Fig. 3.6** Garretson Hospital. FAGGART, HAROLD L., and James E. Garretson. "DR. JAMES E. GARRETSON AND THE FIRST HOSPITAL OF ORAL SURGERY." Bulletin of the History of Medicine 17:4 (1945), Fig. 4 and Fig. 9. © 1945 Johns Hopkins University Press. (Reprinted with permission of Johns Hopkins University)

## References


1. Garretson JE. Surgical education. Dental. Cosmos. 1866;8:186–8.
2. Garretson JE. A system of oral surgery: Being a treatise on the disease and surgery of the mouth, jaws, face, teeth, and associate parts. 4th ed. United Kingdom: JB Lippincott & Company; 1884.
3. Thorpe BL. James Edmund Garretson, A.B., M.D., D.D.S. In: Koch, CRE. In: History of dental surgery: Biographies of pioneer American dentists and their successors. Akron, OH; 1909. p 395–399.
4. Faggart HL, Garretson JE. Dr. James E. Garretson and the first hospital of oral surgery. Bulletin of the history of medicine. 1945;17(4):360–376.
5. Mylonas AI, James E. Garretson: The originator of the term and specialty of oral surgery. Hellenic Archives of Oral & Maxillofacial Surgery. 2019;3:135–9.

# The Profession and Our Dental Colleges. The American Journal of Dental Science. Vol 29, No 8. December 1895. Dr. Truman Brophy

4

Owen Cheng and Michael D. Turner

**Abstract**

Dr. Truman William Brophy (1848–1928) was a luminary in cleft lip and palate repair and a catalyst for dental education reform. He matriculated from the Pennsylvania Dental College and Rush Medical College, an achievement that established Brophy as one of the earliest dual-degree oral surgeons in the United States. In 1886, Brophy successfully performed his first cleft repair surgery. The technique was named the "Brophy Operation" and involved uniting maxillary bones with wire ligatures, followed by meticulous tissue coaptation. Despite criticisms of its traumatic nature, Brophy's innovative technique laid the groundwork for modern cleft repair surgery. Brophy's impact extended beyond surgical innovation. He played a pivotal role in reforming dental education and elevating dentistry's professional stature. Recognizing the imperative for standardized curricula and stringent admission and graduation criteria, Brophy fervently advocated for change. Dr. Truman William Brophy's enduring legacy reverberates through his influence on cleft repair surgery and dental education.

O. Cheng · M. D. Turner (✉)
Division of Oral and Maxillofacial Surgery, Icahn School of Medicine at Mount Sinai, New York, NY, USA
e-mail: yu.cheng@einsteinmed.org; yc3de@virginia.edu; michael.turner@mountsinai.org

**Keywords**

Truman William Brophy · Cleft lip and cleft palate repair · Brophy operation · Dental Education Reform · Orthognathic surgery

## Introduction

The article titled "The Profession and Our Dental Colleges" was published in December of 1985 in *The American Journal of Dental Science*. It was based upon a presentation given to the Illinois Society of Dentistry on the current state of dental education in the United States. In this visionary article, Dr. Brophy called first on a profession-wide reflection on the quality of dental education, acknowledging the accomplishments far in systemizing and progressing dental education standards and how it further needed to evolve to bring the specialty on par with other health care professions. Dr. Brophy's thoughts and opinions on this guided the advancement of dental education so much so that they are still present in the organization of the curriculum and licensure today.

## Truman Brophy

Truman William Brophy (Fig. 4.1) was born on April 12, 1848. He was the son of Canadian immigrants, William Brophy and Amelia



S. R. Aziz, M. D. Turner (eds.), *Classic Papers and Pioneers in Maxillofacial and Oral Surgery*, https://doi.org/10.1007/978-3-031-63246-4_4

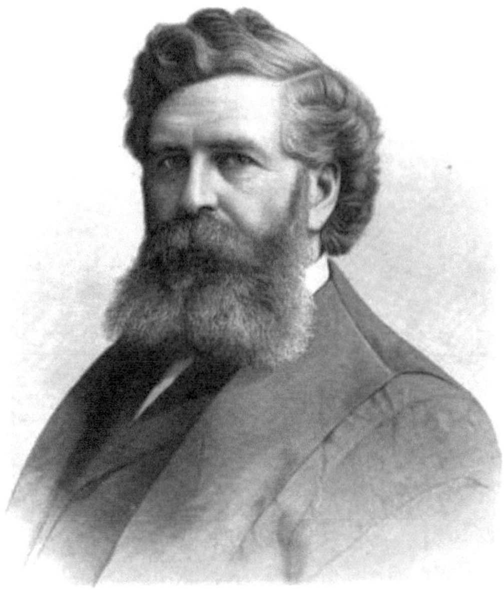

**Fig. 4.1** Dr. Truman William Brophy MD, DDS (1848 –1928)

Cleveland Brophy, and spent his childhood in Illinois on his family's farm. Brophy's first encounter with dentistry was detailed in his memoir, "Brophy, Truman William, and Bertha Robinson. *Truman William Brophy: A Memoir*. Chicago: n.p. 1936":

> When Truman was about twelve years old an itinerant dentist visited his home. The boy was fascinated by the work he saw and the impulse of the moment strengthened into a resolve to become a dentist himself. He was eager to help the visitor in every way he could and, long afterward, in referring to this incident he would say that his first work as a dentist 's assistant was to hold his horse.

This memory greatly influenced the young boy and when Brophy's family relocated to Chicago in the winter of 1866–1867, Brophy immediately sought apprenticeship under the dentist Dr. J. O. Farnsworth. Notably at the time, dental education was in its infantile stages and apprenticeship was the primary pathway toward a career in the field. Brophy's first task as an apprentice was to "manufacture the daily supply of nitrous oxide gas." He learned quickly and within five years, Brophy would succeed Dr. Farnsworth and assume ownership of the practice starting on March 15th, 1871. Unfortunately, the practice was short-lived. Only five months later in October, the infamous Chicago Fires rampaged the city and burned Brophy's newly acquired office to ashes. Wanting to leave the turmoil behind him, and appreciating the importance of formalizing his education, Brophy decided to matriculate into the Pennsylvania Dental College that same fall.

Brophy excelled and graduated the following spring. Soon after, the young dentist would visit several surgical clinics along the east coast in cities like Washington, Baltimore, and New York. Among the doctors that he visited was Dr. Louis Sayre, a prominent orthopedic surgeon in New York. At Dr. Sayre's clinic, Brophy encountered his first cleft lip and palate patient:

> To this clinic, which was large, patients came who suffered from all sorts of deformities, congenital and acquired. On my first visit there was among them a tall, thin, poorly clad woman, bearing all the evidences of extreme poverty. She had brought her little child to the great surgeon with the hope that he might be cured. His deformity was one of the most conspicuous and distressing that ever saddens a home. It consisted in protruding premaxillae, double cleft lip and complete cleft of the palate. The surgeon took the child in his hands and explained to the class the nature of the deformity. He said, in substance, 'Gentlemen: This child's deformity is so extensive, the tissues are so abnormally placed, that it is not amenable to successful treatment—the treatment that would bring all the parts into normal relation. I grasp the child's face with my hand and find that I can move the maxillary bones toward each other. If we had some way by which these bones might be approximated, the premaxillary bones brought into correct contact with the maxillae, immobilize them and bring about a union, we could go far toward correcting the most conspicuous deformity known to mankind. But such an operation has never been performed. We have no way of doing it.'

Challenged by Dr. Sayre's words and with his curiosity piqued, Brophy felt that it was essential to complete a full medical education. As such, in 1878, Brophy enrolled in Rush Medical College and graduated in 1880 as class president. He was immediately appointed the chair of Dental Pathology and Surgery as one of the first dual -degree oral surgeons in United States history. In the following years, Brophy would relentlessly continue his work and research on cleft repair.

## Cleft Lip and Palate Repair

The year 1886 marked a monumental year for Brophy, having successfully performed his first cleft repair surgery with his peers in attendance. His procedure was detailed at the 1893 World's Columbian Dental Congress in Chicago in an address titled "Surgical Treatment of Palatal Defects." While crediting the work of dentists like Dr. La Monier and Dr. Roux, two French dentists who first proposed a cleft palate closure operation, Brophy noted the low success rates and postprocedural functional deficiencies that were often present in these previous operations due to excessive scar tissue and division of musculature. Brophy proposed an alternative method, later to be known as the "Brophy Operation":

> The [...] method of operating upon children younger than three months is to draw the maxillary bones together by means of strong wire ligatures passed through the maxillary bones from the buccal side, where they are secured to lead plates, which act as non-irritant stay attachments. After drawing the bones together so as to close the cleft, the edges of the soft tissues are pared and co-apted with suitable ligatures and the parts maintained until complete union has taken place.
> The advantages claimed for early operations are:
> First—There is less shock experienced by the patient as its nervous and sense organisms are not completely developed.
> Second—The bones are elastic and can be bent without fracture.
> Third—The palatal muscles and other tissues are brought into functional activity and develop normally instead of atrophying.
> Fourth—By uniting the palatal processes of the maxillary bones the teeth develop in proper place for normal occlusion with the teeth of the lower jaw.
> Fifth—In early operations there is less deformity from the adhesions and contractions of scar tissue.
> Sixth—Early operations preclude the habit of acquiring faulty speech.

The method was considered radical for its time, being the one of the first to propose surgery at the early age of under 3 months. Due to the work of British surgeon Dr. Thomas Smith and his use of chloroform as an anesthetic for better control of the surgical field in the 1860s, the age of operation had already drastically dropped from an average of fifteen to three years of age. So, to many within the surgical community, Brophy's proposition to lower the age of surgery even more seemed unnecessary. Conservative treatment through patient education on proper feeding techniques and simply waiting was favored over Brophy's more aggressive stance. Brophy, however, argued that without early intervention, preventable secondary infections of the throat, nose, middle ear, and pharynx were increased. He noted that the bones of infants are also more "elastic" and can be "bent without fracture" during this age, which theoretically improved outcomes. He further added that young babies also felt less pain and thus resulted in less psychological trauma.

More so than the timing of the surgery, Brophy's procedure was most criticized for its traumatic nature. Surgeons such as Dr. James Berry described it as "brutal" due to the extensive fracturing and wiring involved. These condemnations were not without basis. Brophy's method demanded the surgeon to forcibly compress the palatal segments separated by the congenital fissure using lead plates and silver wires inserted through the lateral alveolar bones. As noted by his British contemporary Sir Harold Gillies and many others, "in addition to the tooth buds that may suffer from Brophy's wires, the upper teeth are inclined to be displaced inwards by the operation." Dr. Van Ingen Brown added on to the mounting disparagement, asserting that Brophy's operation caused "serious permanent disfigurement of the nose and face" later in life due to restriction of maxillary growth. Brophy had boldly proclaimed that "no effort [had] been made to trace patients after they left my hands" and thus had little evidence to dispute Brown's claims.

Brophy published his first book in 1915 titled *Oral surgery; A Treatise on Diseases, Injuries and Malformations of the Mouth and Associated Parts*. Then in 1923, Brophy published his second book titled, *Cleft Lip and Palate*, a culmination of his work on cleft repair surgery, head and neck anatomy, and management of cleft lip and palate patients. By the time of his death, Brophy performed over 10,000 cleft repair operations. Despite the controversy surrounding his technique, Brophy's work helped modernize the time frame in which cleft repair surgery should be done on infants.

## Dental Education and Advocacy

Brophy's accomplishments in the field of cleft repair were rivaled in his achievements in modernizing dental education and elevating the field of dentistry. Having experienced the system of both dental apprenticeship and institutional education, Brophy recognized the need to standardize the dental educational curriculum in the United States. He realized that without regulations overseeing schooling and licensing, dentistry would be unable to gain legitimacy in the eyes of the medical and scientific community. His efforts began in 1875 when he appealed to Rush Medical College for the formal establishment of a department of dentistry. The concept was quickly dismissed as dental schools at the time were poorly attended and there was little demand for new institutions.

In fact, dentistry up until the 1800s was primarily seen as a craftsmen's trade and was littered with "quacks" looking to make an easy profit. It was not until the efforts of certain physicians, such as Dr. Horace H. Hayden and Dr. Chapin A. Harris, that dentistry even began being recognized as a necessary and valid medical specialty. As practitioners of dentistry with complete medical training, these doctors would set the groundwork for organized dentistry and dental education. In 1840, Hayden and Harris would go on to establish the first dental school in the United States, the Baltimore College of Dental Surgery. Initial efforts to have the school integrated into the medical program at the University of Maryland failed forcing the two doctors to charter the college as an independent institution. Despite this important milestone, dentistry still faced strong opposition in formalizing its education from both dentists and physicians. Many dentists specifically hoped to maintain the previous system of apprenticeship to profit from the cheap labor their pupils would provide. Physicians, however, simply refused to see dentistry as a respectable and equal profession as medicine. As such, the development of dental schools was sluggish, and attendance was low. By 1865, only four dental schools (including the Baltimore College of Dentistry) remained standing with several others having been discontinued shortly after their inception.

The year of 1867, however, marked a significant landmark in the state of dentistry when Harvard University established a department of dentistry in affiliation with its medical department. For the first time in history, dentistry was given recognition as a field of study through a reputable institution of higher education. Admission requirements, however, were nonexistent and to graduate, students had to successfully complete three years of apprenticeship under a private dentist in addition to two years of the same coursework required of Harvard's medical students.

As the number of graduates from dental schools increased, tensions rose between formally trained dentists and those who learned from the slowly vanishing system of apprenticeship. In effort to legitimize the occupation, organizations such as the American Society of Dental Surgeons were formed, whose goals included giving "character and respectability to the profession, by establishing a line of distinction between the truly meritorious and skillful, and such as riot in the ill-gotten fruit of unblushing impudence and empiricism." This rise of organized dentistry and its political advocacy rapidly brought forth much needed change in the laws regulating dentistry. By 1868, a mere year after Harvard Dental School's inception, the states of New York, Kentucky, and Ohio had passed laws creating official governing bodies to oversee the licensure of legitimate dentists. Such statutes marked the beginning of the end for the system of apprenticeship as states began lawfully requiring a dental diploma as the sole requirement for a license. With the emerging enforcement of these new regulations, dental schools steadily grew in numbers in the following years to accommodate for the increasing number of students. By 1884, approximately twenty-two dental schools had been established with nine being officially associated with a university.

Realizing this change in momentum, Brophy once again appealed to Rush Medical College for the creation of a dental school. His second attempt was successful and in 1883, the Chicago Dental Infirmary was officially chartered. Though originally, the infirmary was intended to train only physicians, this prerequisite was dropped when the school was rechristened as the Chicago College of Dental Surgery a year later in 1884. Brophy, however, held on to this belief of having strict and quality admission requirements for the rest of his educational career. He was instated as the college's dean and soon after inaugurated as Dean Emeritus and President of the Faculty, holding these positions for the remainder of his life.

In that same year, under Brophy's leadership, the Chicago College of Dental Surgery joined the National Association of Dental Faculties (NADF) as one of its founding members. The association, which Brophy later led as president, aimed to "bring about the adoption of a uniform standard of graduation" and included schools such as Harvard University and the Baltimore College of Dental Surgery. Due to the growing demand for dental schools, several entities began taking advantage of these positive sentiments through creating dentals schools for the sole purpose of financial profit. These "diploma mill" schools were often short-lived due to their poor educational standards and stained the reputation of dentists by graduating practitioners of inadequate skill and knowledge. As such, organizations like the NADF were vital in both the preservation and advancement of quality dental education. Though the NADF eventually dissolved, the association made notable changes by increasing the length of curriculum to three years in 1891 and then to four years in 1917.

In 1895, Dr. Brophy spoke on the state of dental education in an address to the Illinois Society titled "The Profession and Our Dental Colleges. The American Journal of Dental Science. Vol 29, No 8. December 1895." Brophy called for a profession-wide reflection on the quality of dental education, first acknowledging the accomplishments thus far in systemizing and progressing dental education standards, particularly those of the NADF:

> The dental colleges of the United States, by concert of action, have advanced the curriculum, so that it is today more systematic than in other professional schools.
>
> The effort of the National Association of Dental Faculties to unify the course of study in the several institutions, while not entirely successful, has brought the colleges closer together in the methods of teaching, and the matter taught, than prevailed before the organization of that body.
>
> The extension of the course of study over a period of three years has made it possible for students to bestow more time on the practical phases of anatomy, histology, bacteriology, chemistry, technology, etc., besides becoming more proficient in operative and prosthetic dentistry. The changing of the course, therefore, from two to three years has not only met with the approval of the profession, but has been equally gratifying to the faculties; so this relation of our colleges to the profession has been most happy.

Despite the improvements to the dental curriculum over the years, admission criteria remained essentially nonexistent and prospective students were not even required to have completed high school. Accordingly, Brophy emphasized the necessity of setting stringent prerequisites to screen for students with "prompt aptitude" who have "already acquired certain fundamental knowledge." His suggestions included even necessitating prospective students complete a "course in manual training school" to build a baseline for "the manipulation of metals, the handling of fine instruments, and the manual dexterity essential to [their] success as a dental practitioner." Brophy ultimately sought out students "with a love for [dentistry] prompted by the desire to excel, not stand among the mediocrity of [their] profession, but with a determination to reach the topmast rung of the ladder of professional fame."

In efforts to continue the legitimization of the dental profession, he further argued that schools should release students unable to meet the educational standards set before them. Brophy asserted that "the duty of the colleges to the profession should be to guard their entrances and their exits; admit only such young men as possess a good education; watch them carefully; advance them practically and scientifically; and in the event of their failure to become skilled in the operating room and laboratories, they should reserve the right to return them their fees pro rata, and advise them to engage in some other vocation." He suggested that the state should also "visit the dental colleges more frequently, and by their presence stimulate the students to make their very best efforts."

With the increasing number of dental schools, however, many private practitioners felt threatened as the more affordable student-run clinics began eroding their patient pools. They complained that schools too often "receive[ed] and perform[ed] operations for persons who are abundantly able to compensate a practitioner for his services." Conversely, Brophy noted that dentists too often extracted teeth that could be restored more conservatively. Tensions were bubbling, which Brophy perceived as an internal threat to the profession's reputation and progress. A mutually beneficial solution was necessitated and so in his address, Brophy proposed the following:

> The colleges should not receive patients who are financially able to compensate dentists for their services. Members of the profession should not extract teeth which are susceptible of being treated and filled, on the ground that the financial condition of the patient will not permit them to spend the necessary time to treat them and put them in a healthy, satisfactory condition, but should, in all such cases, issue a card to such a patient and send him to a college infirmary, where such a card should admit him to treatment.

Brophy ultimately saw the potential of the school clinics to not only provide affordable and proper care but also as an instrument to educate "people up to the value of the teeth and the advantages to be derived by preserving them." He hoped to unify the dental profession by instilling a collective purpose to provide "the public to an appreciation of the great benefits which are bestowed on them by scientific and practical dentistry." With this overarching idea in mind, Brophy ended his address applauding the work of his peers, the Illinois General Assembly, and the Illinois State Board of Dental Examiners for their success in strengthening the profession. However, aware of the dangers of complacency, Brophy cautiously reminded the audience that the law still "has certain defects which should be amended."

In particular, the laws regulating licensure remained much too lax by granting any individual with a diploma, the ability to legally practice regardless of education quality. A standardized board licensing exam was needed to weed out "diploma mill" school graduates. Brophy pointed out that due to such defects, "permanent licenses have been issued by our State Board to young men who have had but a single course of study; and so their further study has been discontinued, and further proficiency has not been acquired."

## Legacy

Due to these laws, the number of dental schools in the United States swelled from 22 to 57 between 1884 and 1900. While many of these were indeed "diploma mill" schools, the laws did ultimately bring upon the end of the unregulated apprenticeship system and by 1920, only 3% of all dentists had been trained under the said system. In the following years, many of the "diploma mill" schools failed as educational requirements increased in large part due to the efforts of Brophy and his contemporaries. In Illinois alone, 22 dental schools lost their charters between 1902 and 1905. Brophy's advocacy for more stringent admission criteria also proved successful and by the 1920s a minimum of a high school diploma was necessary to be admitted.

In 1923, the National Association of Dental Faculties officially dissolved upon joining arms with the Canadian Dental Faculties, the American Institute of Dental Teachers, and the Dental Faculties Association of American Universities to amalgamate as the American Association of Dental Schools (AADS). The congregation of these overseeing organizations symbolized the

AADS's unifying goal "to facilitate intercourse and conference among teachers of the dental sciences and arts in North America; to promote advancement of teaching and research in American schools of dentistry; to encourage thorough study and discussion of the needs and problems of dental education; to improve public understanding and appreciation of the quality and value of dentistry; and to maintain dental education in full accord with the highest requirements of professional education in the public service." Today, the AADS is currently known as the American Dental Education Association (ADEA).

The year 1923 also marked the year in which the Chicago College of Dental Surgery was integrated into Loyola University and renamed as the Loyola University Chicago Dental School. While the school ultimately closed in 1993, Brophy's lifelong efforts and work played an indispensable role in transforming the landscape of dental education.

On February fourth, 1928, Dr. Truman Brophy passed away from pneumonia at the age of 79 in Los Angeles, California. He left behind an enduring legacy in his contributions advancing cleft repair surgery, modernizing dental education, and advocating for the dental profession nationally and globally. During his illustrious career, he served as president for the Illinois State Dental Society, Chicago Dental Society, Odontological Society of Chicago, the National Association of Dental Faculties, and the Fédération Dentaire Internationale. As listed in his memoir, his lifetime honors also include the following:

- *Officer of Public Instruction, France, 1913.*
- *Officer of the Legion of Honor, France, 1924.*
- *The Miller Memorial Prize— Federation Dentaire Internationale, 1925.*
- *"Homenje Al Talento" — a Medal from Professor J. J. Rojo, Mexico City, 1902*
- *William Jarvie Fellowship Medal, The Dental Society of the State of New York (for distinguished services to dentistry), 1906.*
- *Medal for "Merited Distinction" from the Odontological Society of Paris, 1903.*
- *Italian Stomatological Society Medallion, 1913.*

## Further Reading


Berry and Legg. Harelip and cleft palate. London: Churchill; 1912.

Brock C. Surgery, success, and the role of the patient in cleft palate operations, circa 1800–1930. Isis. 2022;113:1.

Brophy TW. Surgical treatment of palatal defects. In: Harland AW, editor. Transactions of the World's Columbian dental congress, vol. 2. Chicago: Press of Knight, Leonard & Co.; 1894. p. 532–50.

Brophy TW. Oral surgery, a treatise on the diseases, injuries and malformations of the mouth and associated parts. Philadelphia: P. Blakiston's Son; 1915.

Brophy TW. Cleft lip and palate. Philadelphia: P. Blakiston's Son; 1923.

Brophy TW, Robinson B. Truman William Brophy: a memoir. Chicago: Children of Truman William Brophy; 1936.

Brown VI. The surgery of oral diseases and malformations, their diagnosis and treatment. Philadelphia: Lea & Febiger; 1912.

Gies WJ. Dental education in the U.S. and Canada: a report to the Carnegie Foundation for the Advancement of Teaching. New York: Carnegie Foundation for the Advancement of Teaching; 1926.

Institute of Medicine (US). Committee on the future of dental education. In: Field MJ, editor. Dental education at the crossroads: challenges and change. Washington, DC: National Academies Press (US); 1995.

Kinsley P. Truman Brophy, famous Chicago surgeon, is dead. Chicago Tribune, February 05, 1928.

Murray RW. The treatment of cleft palate. Lancet. 1911;2:1466–9, on p. 1467.

Owen E. Cleft-palate and hare-lip. London: Baillière, Tindall and Cox; 1904.

Parsons M. Loyola closing dental school. Chicago Tribune, June 9, 1992.

Roberts JB. 1852–1924. Surgery of deformities of the face: including cleft palate. New York: Wood; 1912.

# Matthew H. Cryer. The Status of the Dental Profession. The Dental Cosmos; A Monthly Record of Dental Science. Volume 45, Issue 2. February 1903

5

Nadia Mezghani and Al Haitham Al Shetawi

**Abstract**

In Dr. Matthew H. Cryer's 1903 article titled "The Status of the Dental Profession", he brings attention to a topic that continues to be up for debate more than a century later: the status of the dental profession. Should dentistry be a medical specialty or a profession of its own? Cryer informs the reader of his stance on the issue early on in the article, sharing that he has "no sympathy" for the movement he was witnessing. He argues that the day dentistry becomes a branch of medicine, is the day dentistry will no longer exist. Through Cryer's article, one gets a glimpse of the many debates and arguments that filled much of the dental profession at the time, as some dentists sought to find legitimacy and professionalism by finding a place in the medical profession, while others, such as Cryer, had no intention or desire to do as such. Within this turmoil was the rising field of oral surgery, which one might say, was adding even more fuel to the fire.

N. Mezghani (✉)
Oral and Maxillofacial Surgery, Mount Sinai Health System/Jacobi Hospital, New York, NY, USA

A. H. Al Shetawi
Division of Oral and Maxillofacial Surgery, Head and Neck Surgery, Division of Surgical Oncology, Vassar Brothers Medical Center, Poughkeepsie, NY, USA

**Keywords**

Matthew Cryer · Dentistry · Dental history · Oral surgery

## The Great Debate

The *Dental Cosmos* was the first lasting national journal for the American dental profession and one of the most significant in the early history of American dentistry. The foundation of the dental practice was written and debated in its pages from 1859 to 1836, leading the way as a model of what a successful dental journal could be. The timeless controversy on dentistry's place within the medical world is debated by Dr. Matthew H. Cryer in "The Status of the Dental Profession. The Dental Cosmos; A Monthly Record of Dental Science. Volume 45, Issue 2. February 1903." Cryer's stance on the issue cannot be mistaken as he includes the following statement made by Sir Michael Foster:

> …I venture to think, are agreed that education should be fashioned after the manner of a cone, starting from a broad basis, and narrowing to an apex, for it is the conical bullet that has the penetrating power. In the storm and stress of modern life an all-around education may be good in society, but it is not suited to a profession. The round ball thrown at a surface may make a hole, but it more frequently simply rebounds, whereas the cone may be depended upon to pierce; and the man whose education is conical makes his way. For



S. R. Aziz, M. D. Turner (eds.), *Classic Papers and Pioneers in Maxillofacial and Oral Surgery*,
https://doi.org/10.1007/978-3-031-63246-4_5

> each profession the cone should be different, should be fashioned in different ways, (…) All knowledge is useful, but the power of the human mind to attain and retain knowledge is limited. We cannot all know everything.

The first documentation of dental-related procedures in human history were those pertaining to exodontia, yet these scriptures did not differentiate dentistry from medicine. The divide between the fields of dentistry and medicine in the United States has not always been as we know it today; one will find that the formal place of dentistry in American medical history is much of a gray matter. Despite these deep historical ties with medicine, American dentistry took its own route, from its own schools to its own journals and societies, ever since the early 1800s. Continuing to the present day, there have been both proponents and critics of the mere idea of dentistry and medicine as one. Cryer continues by quoting a speech from the International Dental Federation meeting of 1902:

> Although dentistry was once an intimate part of the medical art, it can hardly be so again, for its evolution has been so complete that it now forms a distinct separate division of the art of healing. It is, I venture to think, a child of the old stock destined to continue an independent existence and to work out its own salvation [1].

## The Early Nineteenth Century and the Financial Panic

The early nineteenth century faced an era of dysregulated dentistry; the field was overrun by unqualified individuals and managed largely as a free-for-all [2]. There were two types of dentists: medical-dentists and craft-dentists. The former learned the practice through apprenticeships from competent providers, while the latter practiced dentistry mainly from a mechanical scope, usually alongside another trade. There was no regulation of practice in place for the public to decipher a competent, professional dentist from an imitator. It was not until 1834 that the first institutionalized group, the Society of Surgeon-Dentistry of the City and State of New York, was formed by a group of 50 reputable dentists.

The financial panic of 1837 was the start of a marking point for the dental profession. With the widespread unemployment rates and lack of a system in place, the number of "dentists" doubled within 2 years [3]. The growing cities and the sought-after urban living of the time increased the demands of the profession. This era not only affected the qualified professionals but also the public's image of the profession itself. There was no professional degree or license for qualified dentists to prove their legitimacy. Any kind of academic degree, no matter how irrelevant, was a dentist's only hope of gaining the public's trust and business. Dentistry was fighting for professional status and trust in a society that simply could not find the means to provide it, and rightly so.

The connotation of dentistry as a trade of the common man surely did not help its reputation from a scientific standpoint in medicine. It is for this reason and others that perhaps dentistry lagged medicine in terms of institutionalization and credibility. Medicine and dentistry faced similar issues in this regard, although they appeared at different times in the development of both professions. It has been stated that dentistry during this period emasculated the movement of medicine during the late 1800s; both professions were fighting for institutionalization. This period in dentistry was marked by a push against the co-existence of providers holding degrees and those without during a time in which medicine was not yet open to specialization and had surely not forgotten the mechanical focus of craft-dentists [3].

## The Turn of the Century

In 1839, the *American Journal of Dental Science* was launched. The following year was also a memorable one for the profession, articulated with a short script taken from a petition to the state of Maryland to establish the first dental learning institution, the Baltimore College of Dental Surgery: "*…the profession* (dentistry), *they may be enabled to practice it, not alone as a mere mechanical art, but upon sound scientific principles, as a regular branch of medicine*" [2].

Many dentists saw an urgent need to embody an institutionalized form of education. However, it is to be noted that the majority supporting this effort were physicians, not dentists; the medical profession welcomed the new school in Baltimore without hesitation. The relationship between physicians and dentists, at this time, would not go on further than collegiate support, however. Prominent dentists, even medically trained ones such as Samuel Fitch and the founder of the Baltimore school, Horace Hayden, made efforts to interest physicians to the practice. However, the medical community still largely practiced in terms of humoral pathology, as opposed to local disease. Physicians saw no clear indication to give attention to dental diseases or disorders as they considered them unimportant to general health. Dental decay was perceived as a local disease needing mechanical interventions and thus did not call for humoral medicine. In a way, dentistry was practicing local disease at a time when medicine had not reached its scientific revolution to accept it. One dentist, in response to protests for dental education in medical school, is said to have sarcastically suggested that *"the author of such a plan, to be consistent, should fill teeth but treat the constitutional causes of dental caries by bleeding, purging, and leeching his patients"* [2]. William J. Gies identified four major characteristics of dentistry that he believed would prevent physicians from ever growing interest in the field:

> The concurrences of these conditions of incapacity for self-repair, incurability by medicinal treatment, ready recovery from the effects of a total loss, and completeness of the functional restoration attainable by acritical replacement, which do not apply collectively to any other part of the body that is supplied with blood and nerves, long seemed an encouragement of medical indifferent to the teeth and dentistry" [4].

Despite a lack of scientific defense, American dentistry was gaining the public's respect and establishing itself as a true profession. From the discovery of anesthesia in 1844 to the introduction of porcelain teeth, and the founding of the American Dental Association in 1859, dentistry was gaining confidence in the accomplishments it had made. Meanwhile, medicine was still juggling with the problems of specialization.

## The Oldest Specialty

Although the history of oral surgery cannot be discussed outside of the context of dentistry, most of the advances in the field originate from surgeons rather than dentists [5]. Most of the specialty's pioneers were trained both in dentistry and medicine, holding dual degrees. Despite this, it is evident that these early pioneers firmly believed that the practice was a branch of dentistry and not medicine. The American pioneers of oral surgery were sprouting the profession at a time when the mouth did not have a place in traditional human anatomy courses, let alone medicine itself [6]. As one of these pioneers himself, Cryer continues in his chapter to say:

> Dentistry in America did not originate from medicine. Scientific dentistry began here as a separate profession in specially established schools he day the degree of Doctor of Dental Surgery was conferred upon by Drs. Arthur and Mackall in 1841 [1].

The introduction of oral surgery as a distinct entity from either general surgery or dentistry added further dispute; medical colleagues were still holding on against the idea of specialties. The appreciation for oral surgery as a distinct field was not given until 1869 when Dr. James Garretson was entitled and appointed Oral Surgeon to the Hospital of the University of Pennsylvania. He had previously joined the Philadelphia Dental College as Professor of Anatomy and Surgery in 1864 and made great efforts to incorporate surgery into the dental curriculum; this was perhaps the first evidence of such teaching, all while still holding the title of "dentist." Garretson was not afraid to show full support for the establishment of oral surgery as a distinct specialty, instructing medically trained dentists to "*go into the American Medical Association not as dentists, but as oral surgeons - as gentlemen of full medical education*" [2]. The Civil War further aided the dental profession in holding on to oral surgery as its own specialty; contributions and advances in facial fractures and trauma made it clear that oral surgery was in the hands of dentists, and not general surgeons.

The argument settled for some time into the later part of the nineteenth century. Each profession went its separate way and it was not until after the close of the century in 1910 that William Hunter, an English physician, read a paper before the Faculty of Medicine of McGill University. Hunter accused dentists of causing disease by creating "*a veritable mausoleum of gold over a mass of sepsis to which there is no parallel in the whole realm of medicine or surgery*" [7]. The theory of focal infection, owing to the rise of bacteriology and the discovery of the X-rays, was soon swept throughout the medical and dental professions.

Into the twentieth century, dentistry sensed the pressure to follow the trajectory of its first specialty and draw itself closer to scientific reasoning if it was to continue being appreciated and respected as more than a mechanical art. It was time for the dental profession to look through the lens of scientific reason, something they had come to under-appreciate, but never fully rejected. It was a lens that had been briefly described but not completely taken into action for almost a century prior:

> At present, a spirit of inquiry is abroad and I cannot, but anticipate a period, when, upon this subject, prejudices shall be removed, malpractices correct, the darkness of ignorance be dispelled, and commensurate with the talents and worth of many of its professors, its extensive bearing upon health, and its happy influence upon society, (dentistry will) assume a correspondent rank among the Medical Sciences.—Samuel S. Fitch, 1829 [8].

## Early Life and Education

Matthew Henry Cryer (Fig. 5.1), son of Henry and Elizabeth (Cookson) Cryer, was born on July 21, 1840, in Manchester, England. At the age of 11, he moved with his family to the United States and 10 years later enlisted in the US Army. Cryer, having joined the sixth Ohio Cavalry, fought in many battles including the battles of the Wilderness, Trevilian Station, Mallory's Cross Roads, and Saint Mary's Church. He was even

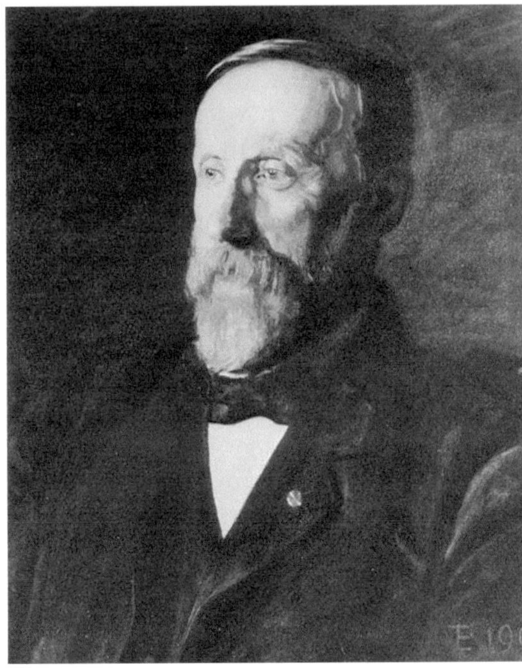

**Fig. 5.1** Painting of Dr. Matthew H. Cryer by Thomas Eakins between circa 1870 and 1910. (Reprinted by The Art of Philadelphia Medicine, Philadelphia Museum of Art, 1965)

wounded at a Battle in Virginia in 1864. The following year, he advanced to the rank of major and took great pride in his service.

After his years in the army, Cryer went on to earn his dental degree in 2 years from the Graduate Philadelphia Dental College in 1876. He then earned his medical degree from the University of Pennsylvania in 1877.

## A Teacher and Futurist

Cryer dedicated over 20 years of his life as a lecturer on mechanical dentistry at the Philadelphia Dental College. Beginning in 1900, he would serve as an oral surgeon on the staff of the Philadelphia Hospital. Apart from this role, he was also a visiting surgeon at the Philadelphia General Hospital and a consulting surgeon at the University Hospital. Cryer was an activist for his profession and continuously sought ways to move his profession forward; he was a member of the Academy of Stomatology, American Dental Society, American Society for the Advancement of Sciences, and the Pathological Society of Philadelphia. Cryer even went on to serve as president of the Pennsylvania State Dental Society in 1902.

Perhaps one of Cryer's most recognized works was related to his commitment and fascination for the human anatomy. Cryer's profound interest led him to publish the book entitled *Internal Anatomy of the Face* in 1901 and a second addition in 1916. For decades, Cryer collected hundreds of skulls, sectioning and precisely studying every one of them (Fig. 5.2).

> This investigation completely overturned the [my] conception of what was meant by the term typical. There is, doubtless, a typical or typal form for each bone, but it is not often found in nature. If we were to photograph a thousand temporal bones, for example, and make a composite of the entire number, the composite would properly be accepted as figuring the typal temporal. It is possible, though doubtful, that of the thousand bones, two or three

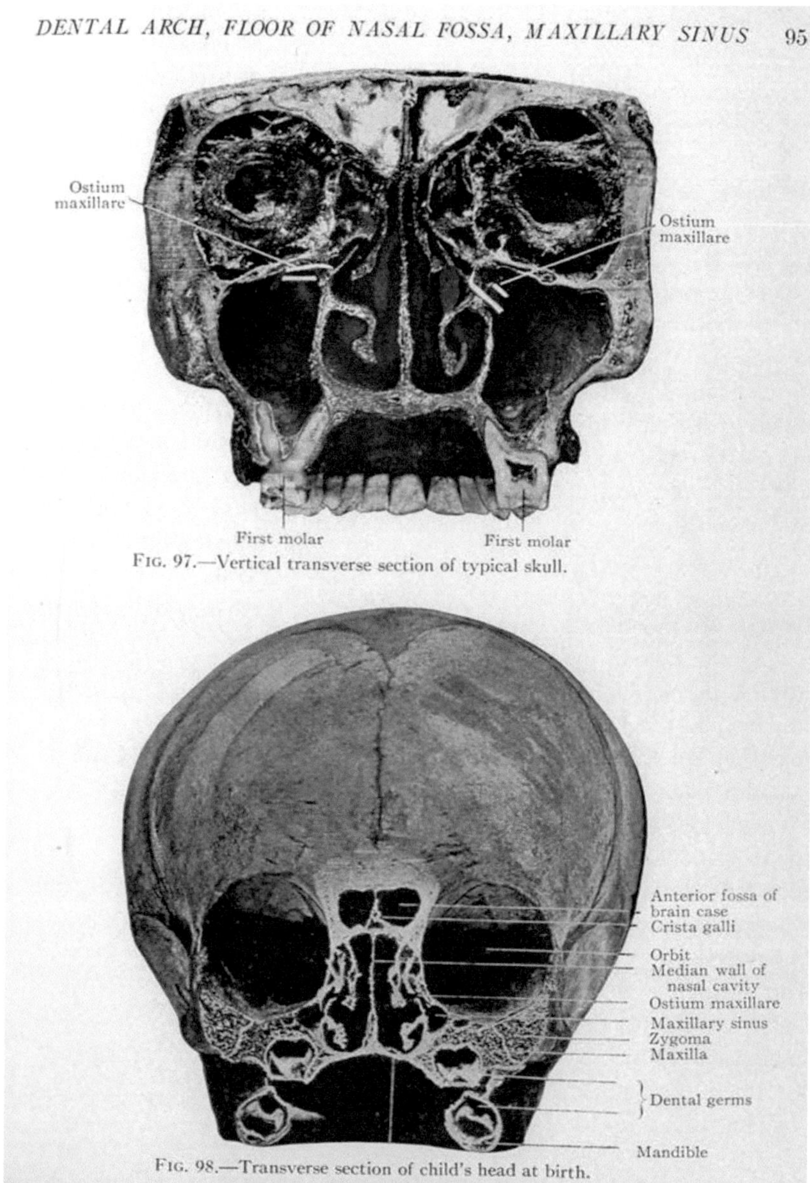


**Fig. 5.2** Illustrations from Dr. Matthew H. Cryer's book, *Internal Anatomy of the Face* [9]

> could be found which would exactly correspond with the typal bone so pictured. This in the writer's view, is strong testimony that the typal bone is ideal; that the actual is a variant. It is with these variants that the surgeon and dentist have practically to deal [9].

Cryer's dedication to uncovering the variations encountered during practice, unlike the standard, textbook anatomy, molded how the profession would be taught and learned for years to come. He once said that "*the study of oral surgery first requires that the oral surgeon shall know minutely the anatomy, physiology, and pathology of the parts of which he is dealing. This means more than one might first suppose, as one cubic inch of the parts associated with the mouth contains more varies tissue than an entire leg*" [10]. Cryer advocated for the "intimate study of the body," and the notion that textbooks should only be a mere supplement to firsthand learning. He advocated that textbooks cannot be used as guides or roadmaps through surgery; textbooks are not any more than general truths. Lack of knowledge of or stubbornness for the variation observed in human facial anatomy, Cryer proposed, is the basis to explain many of the failed operations of his time and not the natural percentage of the unsuccessful treatment. Cryer's collection of specimens and skulls is thought to be one of the largest and most complete in existence and today can be found in the Mutter Museum of the College of Physicians in Philadelphia.

Cryer also holds the title of founding the first hospital-based dental service in 1901 at the Philadelphia General Hospital [11]. The preceding year, Dr. John Shoemaker, president of the Board of Charities and Correction of the City of Philadelphia, acted upon the observation that many patients at the Philadelphia Hospital required dental care. The hospital board soon went on to direct one of the oral surgery staff to begin delivering dental care to these patients. This member was Cryer himself, and he led a small service of three other dentists and two interns into the making of history. As an advocate for teaching and learning, Cryer incorporated teaching clinics for local dental students into the service. The service would now go on to serve two purposes: patient care and student training, which continue to be the basis of dental residency programs today. It was not until 1943 that the American College of Surgeons passed a minimum standard for dental presence in hospitals. Building on Cryer's work, hospital dental services now include administrative, consultation, education, and clinical functions.

From a more technical standpoint, Cryer also made many advances to the instruments used in surgery. In 1904, Cryer designed a pair of universal incisor and root forceps, claiming that they could be used to extract any tooth in the moth. He also redesigned a pair of left and right scaling instruments to be heavier, owing to the development of what is known today as the left and right Cryer elevators. He is also remembered for developing the electrically operated surgical engine and a spiral osteotome with a guard for cranial surgery. Cryer had observed unsuccessful attempts to protect the dura during cranial surgeries. The main difference in his design was that the saw was arranged to cut in a line with the axis of the shaft of the burr, and not at a right angle as the traditional circular saws, allowing for cutting in any direction and upon curved lines (Fig. 5.3) [12]. His addition of a button-like guard at the point of the burr was shown to prevent any injury to the dura, and his design remains the basis of existing devices today.

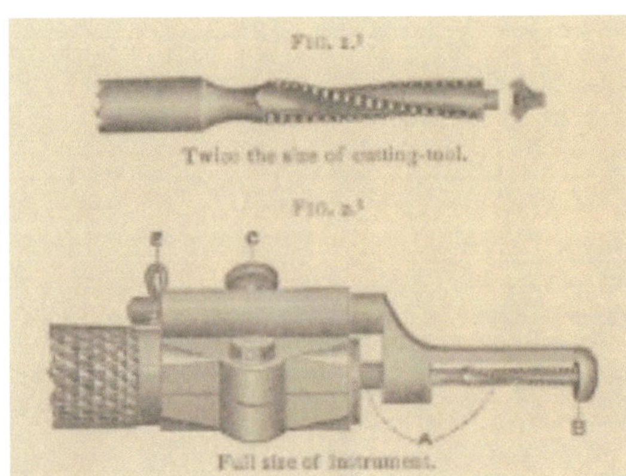


**Fig. 5.3** Sketches of Dr. Matthew H. Cryer's osteotome [12]

## The Legacy

Cryer had a futurist outlook on surgery, during a time when many surgeons were not interested in deviating from the traditional technique and tools; during a discussion about Cryer's device at the Philadelphia Country Medical Society, a physician stated:

With regard to this elaborate instrument, it seems to work satisfactorily, yet for my own work I should rather use a sharp chisel with my own hand and my own mallet than any mechanical device. What we want to do is to train our own hands to do the work, and not be dependent upon any mechanical device" [13]. Cryer argued that surgery would take a step back if mechanical devices were not used, and stated, with good humor, to "not be dependent upon any mechanical device," poses a mere contradiction, since the physician admits to using one himself, "albeit a very crude one, in the shape of a mallet and chisel. I consider this engine as far in advance of chisel and mallet in bone surgery as the Pullman car is ahead of the canal boat in traveling.

Matthew Cryer passed away on the 12th of August in 1921. His emphasis on the variation of human facial anatomy and teaching style pivoted how future oral surgeons were trained, and this legacy is still reflected to this day. Cryer defended his profession, in the lowest and highest of times, and his passion to continue advancing the profession is beautifully articulated in one of his greatest hopes: "*If dentistry be allowed to simply become a specialty of medicine, then the dental profession will cease to exist. This I sincerely hope will never occur. To prevent it we must continue to elevate the dental profession step by step, as the medical and other professions are being elevated.*"

## References


1. Cryer MH. The status of the dental profession. Cosmos. 1903;45(2):101–5.
2. Schwartz LL. The historical relations of American Dentistry and Medicine. Baltimore, MD: The John Hopkins University Press; 1954. p. 28.
3. McCluggage RW. A history of the American dental association: a century of health service. Chicago, IL: American Dental Association; 1959.
4. Gies WJ. Dental education in the United States and Canada. A report to the Carnegie Foundation for the advancement of teaching. J Am Coll Dent. 1926;79(2):32–49.
5. Fry WK. The evolution of Oral surgery. Proc R Soc Med. 1950;44:139.
6. Thoma KH. The history of oral surgery: the oldest specialty of dentistry. Oral Surg Oral Med Oral Pathol. 1957;10(1):1–10.
7. Hunter W. An address on the role of sepsis and of antisepsis in medicine. Lancet. 1911;1:79–86.
8. Fitch SS. A system of dental surgery: in three parts. New York: G. & C. & H. Carvill; 1829.
9. Cryer MH. Internal anatomy of the face. Philadelphia, PA: Lea & Febiger; 1916. p. 2.
10. Cryer MH. The contributions of dentistry to surgery. Dental Cosmos. 1887;39:102–11.
11. Ivy RH. Fifty years of dental service and internship at the Philadelphia General Hospital. Oral Surg Oral Med Oral Pathol. 1952;5(4):335–9.
12. Cryer MH. A spiral osteotome for opening the skull in brain-surgery. The Medical News. 1894.
13. Cryer MH. The surgical engine and its use in bone surgery. Oral Surg. 1915:258–64.

# 6 The Relation of Oral Surgery to Dental Practice. The Dental Cosmos; A Monthly Record of Dental Science. [Vol. 71]/1929, Volume: 71, Issue: 12, December, 1929, pp. 1165–117

Brent B. Ward


**Abstract**

Chalmers J. Lyons, "The Chief" was a pioneering surgeon who established one of the first residency programs in oral and maxillofacial surgery in the nation. His article, "The Relation of Oral Surgery to Dental Practice" sought to address the challenges of the day, many of which remain "not far from us" as a specialty, seeking to blend dentistry and medicine.



**Keywords**

Oral surgery · Dentistry · Medicine


Recently, the University of Michigan celebrated its 100th year of a residency training program in oral and maxillofacial surgery (OMFS). Chalmers J. Lyons, DDS, "The Chief" (Fig. 6.1) established a 1 year residency program in 1917 encouraged

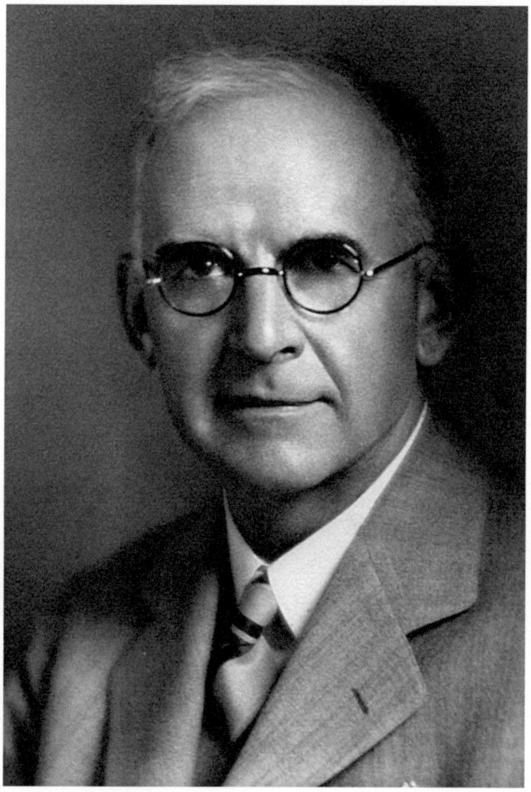

**Fig. 6.1** Portrait of Chalmers J. Lyons, kindly provided by the Chalmers J. Lyons Academy of Oral and Maxillofacial Surgery

by Cyreneus Darling, MD, Chief of Surgery at the University of Michigan Hospital. Dr. Lyons was a pioneer in oral surgery paving the way to


B. B. Ward (✉)
Department of Oral and Maxillofacial Surgery/Hospital Dentistry, School of Dentistry, Ann Arbor, MI, USA

Section of Oral and Maxillofacial Surgery, Department of Surgery, Michigan Medicine, Ann Arbor, MI, USA

Chalmers J. Lyons Academy, Ann Arbor, MI, USA
e-mail: bward@umich.edu





S. R. Aziz, M. D. Turner (eds.), *Classic Papers and Pioneers in Maxillofacial and Oral Surgery*,
https://doi.org/10.1007/978-3-031-63246-4_6

the specialty we enjoy today. His article "The Relation of Oral Surgery to Dental Practice" was read before the Dental Society of the State of New York in 1929 more than 10 years after establishing the residency. The article tenants are indicative of the challenges of establishing and defining the practice of oral surgery in those early days as well as attempting to clarify some of the early misgivings related to teeth and systemic disease.

Based on documented history, the first trainees of Dr. Lyons experienced many challenges being understood and recognized as a profession in hospitals. While the American Association of Exodontists existed, its membership was small and controversial. In reviewing his paper, one must acknowledge that many of the concepts he espoused were not only true then but remain true today as driving principles in educating dental students and OMFS residents. While techniques of surgery have dramatically changed, the field of OMFS remains a bridge between medicine and dentistry as suggested by Dr. Lyons. Oral and Maxillofacial Surgery at the University of Michigan has long been highly regarded among its physician colleges. In 1998, the author accepted the opportunity to be the first OMFS resident to enter dual training in medicine completing his OMFS training in 2000 concurrent with first and second years of medical school and his MD requirements in 2001, followed by a dual two-year certificate in general surgery and a certificate in oral/head and neck oncology. Today, while the Department of Oral and Maxillofacial Surgery/Hospital Dentistry is housed in the School of Dentistry, OMFS faculty in the medical center are dual appointed in the School of Medicine as a section in the Department of Surgery; a true blend of training and appointment alluded to in the visionary statements of Chalmers J. Lyons himself in the article reviewed.

Dr. Lyons believed that oral surgery was simply "general surgery of the oral cavity" drawing on the same principles of surgical practice. Additionally, that the mouth should be viewed as "a part of the whole body" suggesting the importance of a broad medical understanding for dentists. He quotes Dr. Charles May in suggesting a broad view and recognition that the oral cavity can be a causative agent of systemic disease or the recipient of systemic disease abnormalities.

Dr. Lyon's promoted the idea of the need for knowledge in medicine and dentistry. He further denoted that the "dentist of today is able to talk the same language as the physician" and that, "Dentistry must become impregnated with the idea that health conservation is just as important if not more so than tooth conservation."

In his paper, Dr. Lyons goes on to describe root resection, alveolectomy preparatory to denture construction, infections of the maxillary sinus, extractions and acute infections with a concluding statement that "good minor oral surgery must be practiced more extensively by the general practitioner". It is clear that while the focus of the paper was on minor surgery that his practice at the time included clefts and fractures which was somewhat a confusion to the physicians of the time.

A SHORT BIOGRAPHY OF CHALMERS J. LYONS was penned by U.G. Rickert and John W. Kemper.

Doctor Chalmers J. Lyons represented a type of personality that could have served well in any profession. The inspiration that he has given will continue to live. His counsels will always guide those of us who knew him best.

Doctor Lyons was born in Martinsburg, Ohio, April 30, 1874. He was the son of John P. and Manila (White) Lyons. At the age of seven, he came with his family to a farm near Mt. Pleasant, Michigan. It was in the rural schools and at the Central State Normal College at Mt. Pleasant that he received his early education. A descendant of a long line of school teachers, he himself at the early age of 16 also took up this vocation.

After finishing the normal school, he decided to study dentistry. His big problem was how to finance this. Few of us knew that Doctor Lyons was also a pen artist. With this talent and the ability he had, as a salesman, he traveled from town to town taking orders of business men from the blacksmith to the haberdasher for an artistically designed directory. This directory was neatly and attractively penned and framed by the skilled young artist. Hanging in public places, it served not only as a directory but also as creditable advertising.

After Doctor Lyons had covered a considerable part of the lower peninsula of Michigan, he crossed the river and went into Ontario where he was equally successful. He occasionally reminisced with his friends of his experiences, accompanied by Doctor O. W. White of Detroit, in this Canadian business venture. Sufficient funds were thus earned so that he was able to attend the University of Michigan School of Dentistry from which he received the degree of Doctor of Dental Surgery in 1898 and the degree of Doctor of Dental Science in 1911.

In 1907, he moved to Jackson, Michigan, where he became associated in general practice with his brother, Dr. J. W. Lyons. In 1909, he was married to Grace B. Driggs of Palmyra, Michigan. Their son, Richard Hugh, is now a senior in the Medical School of the University of Michigan.

From 1907 to 1909, Doctor Lyons was an instructor in Clinical Dentistry at Ann Arbor. In 1910, he became non-resident lecturer on Clinical Dentistry. In 1911, he was given the post-graduate degree of Doctor of Dental Science. From 1913 to 1915, he served as instructor in Oral Surgery and Consulting Dental Surgeon to the University Hospital.

Doctor Lyons took special instruction in cleft lip and cleft palate surgery from the late Doctor Truman Brophy of Chicago. Following this, he began the notable task of building up the largest clinic of its kind in existence, to which many surgeons came from all parts of the world to observe his methods. In this pioneering work, he had the cooperation of the late Doctors de Nancreed and Cyreneus Darling of the Surgery Department of the University Hospital.

He was made, Professor of Oral Surgery and Consulting Dental Surgeon to the University Hospital in 1915 and continued in this capacity until his death. During the past year, he was made Chairman of the Executive Committee of the School of Dentistry, a position for which he was eminently qualified.

He was active through a most important developmental period of the dental profession and only those of us who knew him best and who observed the keenness with which he could look into the future and analyze situations with the probable outcome can adequately appreciate the tremendous contribution that he made to the recent phenomenal advancement of dental science.

Doctor Lyons' chief ambition was to serve. His skill and ability would have permitted him to capitalize on his services, but not so with Doctor Lyons. He recently made the statement that the most satisfying compensation that he ever had was to see those youngsters upon whom he had operated in babyhood return in him years later to let him see the satisfactory results of the operations. The appreciative mothers who came back to him with the children whom he may have operated as much as 5 or 6 years earlier brought him the type of compensation that gave Doctor Lyons his happiest moments.

He was a frequent contributor to dental and medical literature. He was author of a textbook on "Fractures and Dislocations of the Jaws," and chapters in Ward's "American Textbook of Operative Dentistry" and Mead's "Oral Surgery."

Despite his busy life, Doctor Lyons found time to participate actively in many organizations. He was a member of the American Medical Association, American Dental Association, American Association of Oral and Plastic Surgeons, International Association for Dental Research, Fellow of the American College of Dentists, and Michigan State Advisory Council of Health. He was also a member of Sigma Xi, Phi Kappa Phi, Omicron Kappa Upsilon, and Delta Sigma Delta fraternities. He served as President of the American Association of Oral and Plastic Surgeons and the Michigan State Dental Society, also a Supreme Grand Master of Delta Sigma Delta fraternity. In 1933, he was awarded the Jarvie Medal given by the New York State Dental Society for outstanding dental service. Among the many honors that came to him the one which probably gave him the most personal satisfaction was the founding of the Chalmers J. Lyons club, an organization founded in his honor and made up of men who have served a three-year internship under him in the Department of Oral Surgery.

From the Journal of the Michigan Dental Society 1935

"Michigan dentists mourn the passing of their most beloved dentist, their most useful dentist and their most illustrious dentist." These words from the cover page are not mere sentimental exaggerations permitted at a time of bereavement, they are literally and accurately true.

There has been no time for many years when an expression of the leadership of Michigan dentistry as well as of the rank and file, would not have been practically unanimous in placing Dr. Lyons in all three classifications. The only dissenting opinion would have been from Chal, himself, as he was familiarly known.

These facts in themselves tell the story of a rare combination of qualities. It is not often that the most popular man in the profession is also the most useful and most noted. But the popularity was not a studied effort to win acclaim, it came naturally from a kindliness and sympathy and genuine interest. He was never too busy to see the lowliest seeking his help, and he put everyone at ease by a word or look that inspired confidence and esteem. He was the most useful dentist because of his well-known tact and judgment and influence. He was not impulsive and his judgment was considered unusually sound. Consequently he was much sought as a counselor on important dental affairs and his exceptionally wide acquaintance and tact made him an invaluable ally.

His charm of personality as well as skill as an oral surgeon easily made him Michigan's most illustrious dentist. His fame as a surgeon had reached national and international proportions especially in the field of plastic surgery.

Because he occupied such an unusual place in Michigan dentistry, we believe it fitting to devote a considerable portion of this issue to a memorial and in addition to a biographical sketch we have asked a number of friends and co-workers to contribute short articles from various viewpoints.

In doing this we have confined our requests to Michigan residents, well knowing that scattered far and wide are many who would have considered it a privilege to add their word of tribute. But we would not have known where to begin or where to stop and consequently have not gone outside at all.

It is worthy of note to mention here that Chalmers J. Lyons was in fact the father of this Journal, for it was during his term as President of the Michigan State Dental Society in 1918–1919, and by his recommendation that a quarterly Bulletin was first published by the Society. As usual, he laid a wise foundation. The quarterly expanded to a monthly and later to the status of a Journal.

We are sure that we voice the sentiment of the entire membership when we extended to the bereaved wife, son and relatives the sincerest sympathy of the Michigan State Dental Society.

The author acknowledges the generous use of historical contributions and copied verbatim with permission from the achieves of the Chalmers J. Lyons Academy (Fig. 6.2). See cjlyons.org, Heritage.

**Fig. 6.2** Logo of the academy honoring Chalmers J. Lyons legacy

# 7 Report of a Case of Double Resection for the Correction of Protrusion of the Mandible. *The Dental Cosmos*. Volume 48, Issue 8, August, 1906, Pages 817–820

Daniel J. Meara

**Abstract**

Dr. Vilray Papin Blair, born in 1871, was one of the founders of plastic surgery as a specialty and was known for innovation in surgery and excellence in surgical education. Further, in 1908, he spent time with Dr. Edward Angle, legendary orthodontist, studying jaw deformities and though he was not the father of orthognathic surgery, he was a key contributor in the early evolution of the treatment of mandibular prognathism. In 1912, he authored *Surgery and Diseases of the Mouth and Jaws*, which is considered to be one of the first definitive textbooks for oral and maxillofacial surgery and Dr. Blair was a prolific writer, sharing his thoughts and techniques in the advancement of surgery, such as with the 1906 publication, *Report of a Case of Double Resection for the Correction of Protrusion of the Mandible*, an early editorialization on management of the prognathic mandible.

**Keywords**

Dr. Vilray Papin Blair · Dentofacial deformity · Malocclusion · Double resection · Mandibular protrusion · Surgical correction · Orthognathic surgery · St. Louis Missouri

Dr. Vilray Papin Blair, born in 1871, was one of the founders of plastic surgery as a specialty and was known for innovation in surgery and excellence in surgical education (Fig. 7.1). Further, in 1908, he spent time with Dr. Edward Angle, legendary orthodontist, studying jaw deformities and though he was not the father of orthognathic surgery, he was a key contributor in the early evolution of the treatment of mandibular prognathism. In 1912, he authored *Surgery and Diseases of the Mouth and Jaws*, which is considered to be one of the first definitive textbooks for oral and maxillofacial surgery and Dr. Blair was a prolific writer, sharing his thoughts and techniques in the advancement of surgery, such as with the 1906 publication, Report of a Case of Double Resection for the Correction of Protrusion of the Mandible, an early editorialization on management of the prognathic mandible [1].

> The operation was performed December 19, 1897. The subject of operation was twenty-two years of age, of good personal and family history, apparently inclined to be serious and diffident. These traits, I believe, could be partially traced to the

D. J. Meara (✉)
Department of Oral and Maxillofacial Surgery and Hospital Dentistry, Christiana Care Health System, Wilmington, DE, USA

Department of Physical Therapy, University of Delaware, Newark, DE, USA
e-mail: dmeara@christianacare.org



S. R. Aziz, M. D. Turner (eds.), *Classic Papers and Pioneers in Maxillofacial and Oral Surgery*,
https://doi.org/10.1007/978-3-031-63246-4_7

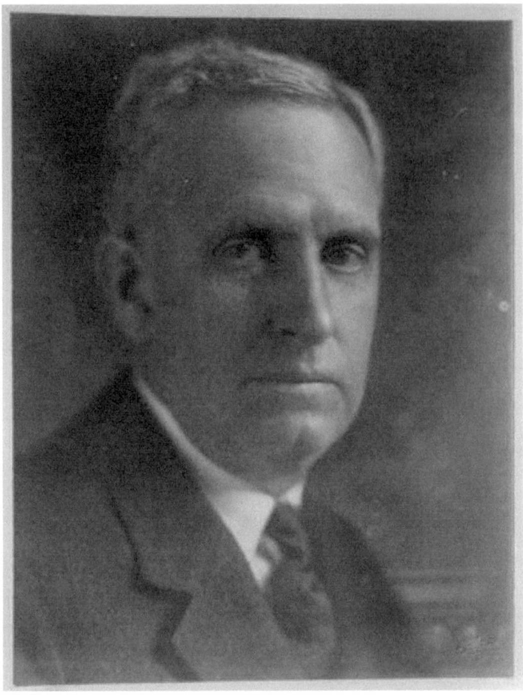

**Fig. 7.1** Portrait of Dr. Vilray P. Blair (1871–1955)

> facial deformity. Some time between puberty and twenty-one years a bilateral growth had occurred in the length of the horizontal ramus of the mandible in one place on each side; that on the left side was between the first and second bicuspid, with a space of one-fourth of an inch between the crowns; that on the right was between the bicuspids and the molar, and was not as great. There was no special separation between the other teeth. The lower third molar articulated squarely with the upper first molar, showing that the mental protrusion was not entirely due to the growth, but that the whole of the tooth-bearing portion of the mandible was in mesial occlusion. There was also a marked lingual inclination of the incisors, the direct result of pressure of the orbicularis oris upon these very prominent teeth. This together with the angling at the site of the abnormal inter-dental spaces produced an obliquity of the chin, so that while the lower incisors were but one-fourth of an inch in front of the upper incisors, the lower mental border protruded much farther.

Dr. Blair believed that the goal of surgery was to: (1) shorten the horizontal ramus and (2) change the mental angle via the removal of excess bone. However, he had questions and concerns regarding the execution of his plan, specifically: (1) could the excess bone be cut-out satisfactorily, (2) would structures in the anterior mandible, specifically, the "inferior dental nerve" be damaged, and (3) could bone growth recur. Dr. Blair pre-surgically addressed these concerns in a variety of ways. The technical removal of excessive bone and the impact on local structures was satisfactorily simulated with experiments upon cadavers and the remaining question regarding regrowth was addressed with the understanding that additional growth and development in a 22-year-old patient was unlikely to occur. Further, Dr. Blair discussed this case with colleagues who concurred with his assessment and surgical plan and the patient decided to have the operation performed, after consultation, due to significant concerns around difficulty eating and speaking. As an aside, prior to surgery the patient was placed into an "apparatus," by his dentist, Dr. Whipple, designed Dr. Edward Angle but apparently "not with the latter's sanction" and was employed in a young adult and not a growing patient, which dismayed Dr. Blair.

> Under chloroform anesthesia, both the head and mandible were held by the hands. I have devised for the bone cuts a double-bladed saw. The skin on the under surface of the chin at a point corresponding to the intended bone cuts was drawn slightly up on the face, and an incision five-eighths of an inch long was made along the outer inferior edge of the horizontal ramus. The result of this skin-drawing was that, when released, the wound slipping back under the chin rendered the scar almost invisible. When the first double cut extended three-fourths of the way through, a similar incision was made on the opposite side. With a rapid mechanical drill, holes for wiring were made near the inferior border of the bone, the saw was replaced, and the sections completed. The mental portion of the mandible was now perfectly movable. Copper wire was passed through the drill holes and the bones were drawn together. This procedure when properly carried out corrects lateral as well as forward protrusion.

Dr. Blair then wired the teeth together, creating a superior tension band at the osteotomy sites and the mandible was placed into the maxilla, for intermaxillary fixation, further "splinting" the mandible to facilitate immobility and ultimately, healing. The documents indicate that the OR case was completed in one hour and ten minutes and the patient required no intraoperative opiates or sedatives. However, several hours after emerging from anesthesia, the patient vomited a significant amount of mucus and blood, which resulted in the patient being released from maxillomandibular fixation. Dr. Blair goes onto recount how the next step in patient management was an error, as the patient was placed into a Barton's bandage of plaster in lieu of replacing the wires for maxillomandibular fixation.

The patient was placed on a "fluid drawn" diet and the recovery was uneventful until the "occurrence of the second accident." Due to patient intolerance and worry, the plaster bandage was removed and it appeared to Dr. Blair that there was bony union on the right side and slight residual motion on the left side. Thus, Dr. Blair asked the patient's dentist, Dr. Whipple to place two dental bands with a bar between them crossing the weak osteotomy site, applying support for continued healing without other means of stabilizing the mandible. Of note, this was the first official consultation with Dr. Whipple by Dr. Blair himself.

> The bands were placed upon the teeth contiguous to the weak section, and through rings on the outer side of these bands a bar was placed that had on it a continuous thread to carry the nuts that held it in place. In drawing on these nuts, the force caused a separation, and there was union on neither side. Dr. Whipple broke the union of the provisional callus. The plaster was reapplied and Dr. Whipple also applied properly adjusted buckles and after several weeks the union was again affected. He also crowned the lower teeth posterior to the cut so that they would occlude with the upper, and filed some points to improve the occlusion of the incisors.

Interestingly, while Dr. Blair was out of the country, Dr. Whipple made a report of this case in *Dental Cosmos*, though he was not present at the operation and lacked details and accuracy in his case discussion which Dr. Blair references as "untrue" and "misleading" in his own *Dental Cosmos* publication of the case and its learnings. Regarding the learnings of the case, Dr. Blair reports that the only long-lasting abnormality was the "complete loss of cutaneous sensation in the lower lip…the sensation of the tooth-pulp is good." Further, the report includes casts to demonstrate the stages of occlusion (Fig. 7.2): (a) represents the casts of the patient's jaws before the operation, (b) shows the early postoperative occlusion after the molars were capped with gold crowns, and (c) shows the potential final occlusion after proper orthodontic treatment. Dr. Blair admits that at the time of the surgery and initial postoperative course, that he did not possess a "proper knowledge of the subject" but that the attention the case garnered fueled his interest to "go deeply into the subject of facial deformities resulting from mal-relation of the jaw-bones." Further, in his subsequent textbook, Dr. Blair cautions the surgeon that

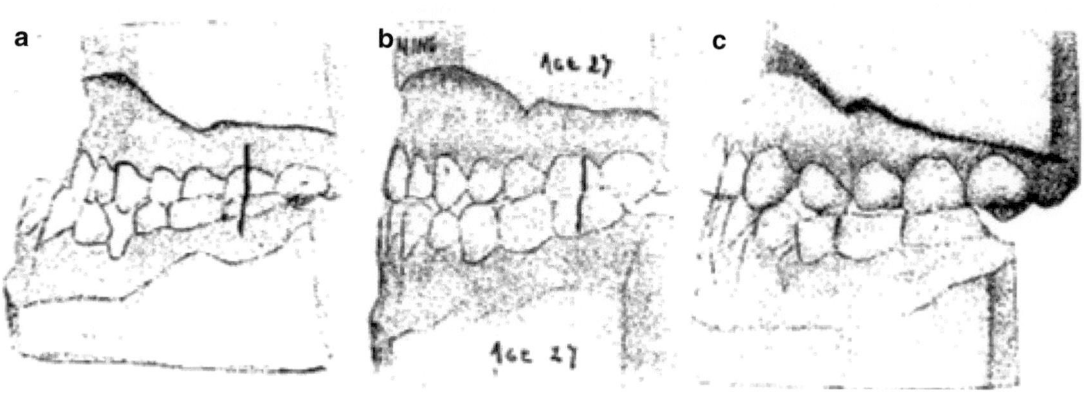


**Fig. 7.2** Case models for patient: (**a**) represents the casts of the patient's jaws before the operation, (**b**) shows the early postoperative occlusion after the molars were capped with gold crowns, and (**c**) shows the potential final occlusion after proper orthodontic treatment

"the lower jaw should be set back only far enough to be in harmony with the rest of the face" and that the surgeon should "leave it to the orthodontist to bring forward the upper incisors if necessary." He stated that "an orthodontist should be involved in the planning of the patient's treatment from the beginning." For some patients, Dr. Blair notes that "it would be of considerable advantage to have the upper jaw, orthodontically, expanded and the upper incisors and canines brought forward before the lower jaw is surgically set back."

Dr. Blair's pioneering work advanced the field of dentofacial deformity correction and was an iterative step building on famous predecessors such as Dr. Simon Hullihen. Also, his willingness to publish, educate others, and seek surgical advancements resulted in enhanced facial surgical patient care throughout the United States and formalized the specialty of plastic surgery while collaborating with dentists, orthodontists, and oral and maxillofacial surgeons.

The story of Dr. Vilray Papin Blair began in St. Louis, Missouri, on June 15, 1871. Dr. Blair was a descendant of the Papins, one of the original French families to migrate to the United States. Further, Dr. Blair was born into a financial well-to-do family, with a grandfather, two uncles, and a father-in-law who were all physicians. His formal early education was elite and he attended Christian Brother's College in St. Louis for his undergraduate college, earning a Bachelor of Arts in 1890 and a Master of Arts in 1894. Thereafter, Dr. Blair attended St. Louis Medical College, but only for one year due to an early interest in engineering at Westinghouse Engineering School. Fortunately for medicine and surgery, his family persuaded him to return to his medical school education. After medical school, he embarked on a 2-year surgical preceptorship at Mullanphy Hospital in St. Louis. This preceptorship stimulated an interest in anatomy that led to Dr. Blair becoming an anatomy instructor at Washington University until 1897, when he traveled to England to study the head, neck, and oral cavity. However, the cost of travel left him in need of a job, and thus, he worked in small health clinics and after one year of surgical training, he became the surgeon for the African Royal Mail Steam Ship Company in London, during expeditions to South America and Africa. As a result of this job, he fought as a troop surgeon with the British Army in 1900 and continued until 1902, when he was appointed to the faculty, as associate professor of surgery and anatomy, at Washington University in St. Louis, MO. As faculty, for the next 6 years, he focused on head and neck reconstructive surgery. Then in 1908, he took a sabbatical to study the management of dental injuries with Dr. Edward Angle, where he advanced surgical technique around the care of mandibular prognathism, including new techniques for mandibular osteotomies. This sabbatical led to Dr. Blair authoring the first definitive text on the treatment of oral–maxillofacial diseases, *Surgery and Diseases of the Mouth and Jaws* as well as subsequent publications on oral surgery topics (Fig. 7.3) [2].

In a form of serendipity, the 1909 Flexner Report for The Rockefeller Foundation on the state of medical training in America, coupled to the presence of Robert H. Barnes, a wealthy businessman in St. Louis, led to the union of Washington University and Barnes Hospital, resulting in one of the most well-funded, progressive academic medical centers in the United States, which bolstered and supported Dr. Blair's forward-thinking surgical concepts and treatments. Another major event that augmented Dr. Blair's skill and knowledge was his wartime experience, as the lead physician for head and neck trauma, in World War I. Upon return from the World War I, at Walter Reed Hospital in DC, Dr. Blair formed a large multidisciplinary team for the care of complex maxillofacial injuries, including dentistry, oral surgery, otolaryngology, ophthalmology, and neurosurgery. This particular team of Dr. Blair's led to the generalized concept of "team care," which spread throughout the United States and the world and resulted in the luminary, Dr. Robert Ivy, creating the first cleft lip and palate team, which is now the standard of care.

Dr. Blair eventually became one of the first non-oral surgeons to be elected to the American Association of Oral and Plastic Surgery

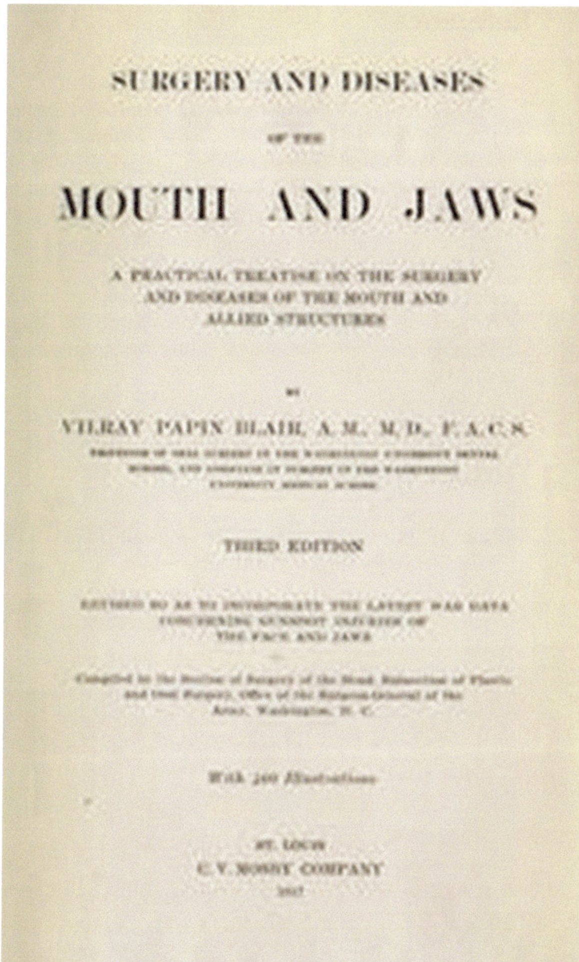

SURGERY AND DISEASES
OF THE
MOUTH AND JAWS

A PRACTICAL TREATISE ON THE SURGERY
AND DISEASES OF THE MOUTH AND
ALLIED STRUCTURES

BY

VILRAY PAPIN BLAIR, A.M., M.D., F.A.C.S.

THIRD EDITION

ST. LOUIS
C.V. MOSBY COMPANY

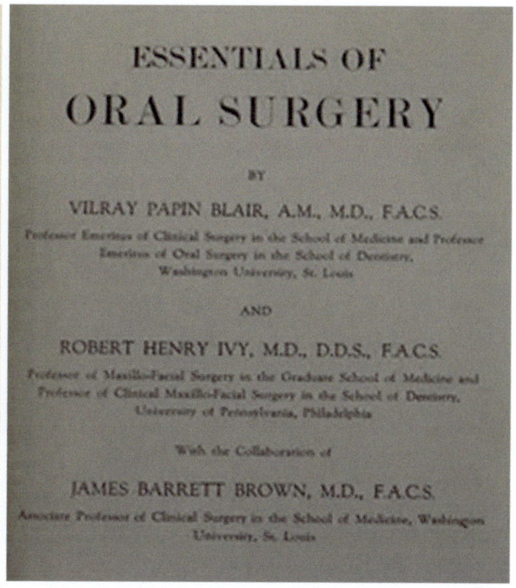

ESSENTIALS OF
ORAL SURGERY

BY

VILRAY PAPIN BLAIR, A.M., M.D., F.A.C.S.
Professor Emeritus of Clinical Surgery in the School of Medicine and Professor Emeritus of Oral Surgery in the School of Dentistry, Washington University, St. Louis

AND

ROBERT HENRY IVY, M.D., D.D.S., F.A.C.S.
Professor of Maxillo-Facial Surgery in the Graduate School of Medicine and Professor of Clinical Maxillo-Facial Surgery in the School of Dentistry, University of Pennsylvania, Philadelphia

With the Collaboration of

JAMES BARRETT BROWN, M.D., F.A.C.S.
Associate Professor of Clinical Surgery in the School of Medicine, Washington University, St. Louis

**Fig. 7.3** Prominent early publications. Top, Surgery and Diseases of the Mouth and Jaws; Bottom, Essentials of Oral Surgery

(AAOPS). Initially, the association was composed of dual degree surgeons (M.D./D.D.S.) interested in diseases of the mouth and jaws. However, eventually the dental degree requirement was discontinued, and the association name was changed to the American Association of Plastic Surgeons, which then led to Dr. Blair helping to form the American Board of Plastic Surgery (ABPS), which provided oversight regarding standards in residency training and faculty qualifications, including scope of practice in the evolving specialty. Regarding scope of practice, Dr. Blair stated that the specialties scope "extended from the top of the head to the soles of the feet," and he was personally at the cutting edge of care for burn victims, cancer patients, dentofacial deformity correction, and cleft surgery.

Lastly, as an anatomist and surgeon, Dr. Blair had an artistic flair that impacted his operating room. Specifically, he engaged Austrian-born, Gisella Loeffler, who studied art at Washington University and became a prominent member of the St. Louis Art Guild, to decorate his operating room in Barnes Hospital, as a calming influence on patients (Fig. 7.4) [3].

Blair died on November 24, 1955, at the age of 84, leaving behind a cadre of trainees that went on to impact surgery and clinical care for decades to come.

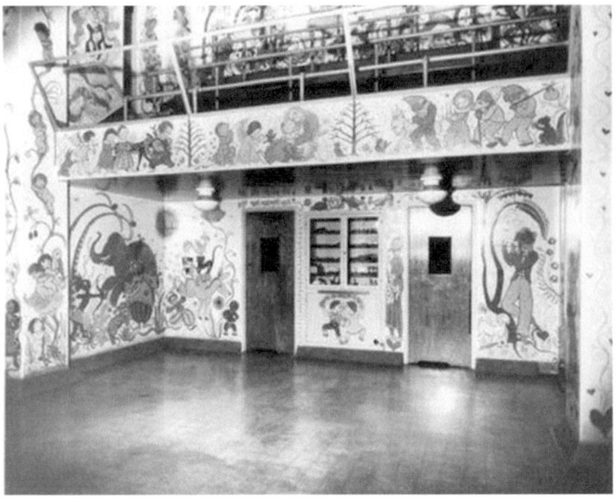

**Fig. 7.4** Dr. Vilray P. Blair's plastic surgery amphitheater in the Rand-Johnson surgical wing at Barnes Hospital was specially decorated by artist Gisella Loeffler, so that young patients would find it less intimidating

## References

1. Blair VP. Report of a case of double resection for the correction of protrusion of the mandible. Dental Cosmos. 1906;48(8):817–20. (now Journal of the American Dental Association).
2. Stelnicki EJ, Young VL, Francel T, Randall P. Vilray P. Blair, his surgical descendants, and their roles in plastic surgical development. Plast Reconstr Surg. 1999;103(7):1990–2009.
3. Becker Archives Database at Washington University School of Medicine in St. Louis. Vilray P. Blair Photographs and Drawings. https://beckerarchives.wustl.edu/VC001.

## Further Reading

Webster JP. In memoriam Vilray Papin Blair, 1871-1955. Plast Reconstr Surg. 1956;18(2):83–112.

# Displacement of the Inter-Articular Cartilage of the Lower Jaw, and It's Treatment by Operation. The Lancet. 1887. Vol 8, pp. 411

8

Michael Proothi

**Keywords**

TMJ · Oral surgery · Jaw surgery · Mandible · Meniscus

Surgical correction of temporomandibular joint disorders is an important and challenging topic in oral and maxillofacial surgery. However, this particular area of our field continues to be controversial. The temporomandibular joint is a complicated anatomic structure of the musculoskeletal system that continues to be treated by many as if it does not exist. On the contrary, treatment approaches have been described through history for over a thousand years including the Hippocratic method of reducing a dislocated mandible [1]. Documented success in surgical management of TMJ disorders has been published in peer-reviewed journals since the 1800s. There is no shortage of TMJ patients seeking treatment, and most are successfully managed conservatively, without surgical intervention. However, patients that can benefit from a surgical procedure have much to gain from a long history of research and clinical validation. This is no different than the surgical management of other synovial lined joints in the body including the hip or the knee. In every aspect of surgery, there is an evolution of procedures which coincides with advances in medicine and biomedical engineering. And we as TMJ surgeons have had our failures, but we have also had significant successes. The first convincing description of successful TMJ surgery was documented in the literature in 1887 by a prominent Scottish surgeon, Dr. Thomas Annandale. His groundbreaking work was published in *The Lancet*.

*The Lancet* is one of the oldest peer-reviewed medical journals in existence. This publication originated in England and has served the medical community with integrity and excellence in engineering, science, medicine, and technology since 1823.

In 1887, at the age of 49, a well-known Scottish surgeon published his TMJ surgical findings in *The Lancet*. The article is entitled: "Displacement of the Inter-Articular Cartilage of the Lower Jaw, and it's Treatment by Operation." Dr. Thomas Annandale was already an accomplished surgeon with several publications and notable professional achievements which will be outlined below. This specific work explored one of the first operative techniques used to correct an intracapsular temporomandibular joint disorder.

> Relaxation the ligaments of the joint allowing a too free movement…..the inter-articular cartilages of the temporo-maxillary joint may become displaced

M. Proothi (✉)
Division of Oral and Maxillofacial Surgery, Department of Hospital Dentistry, Stony Brook University Medical Center, Stony Brook, NY, USA
e-mail: drproothi@stonybrookoralsurgery.com



S. R. Aziz, M. D. Turner (eds.), *Classic Papers and Pioneers in Maxillofacial and Oral Surgery*,
https://doi.org/10.1007/978-3-031-63246-4_8

> either from a sudden tearing of their connexions or from a gradual stretching of them.

In contemporary literature, these words parallel an anteriorly displaced TMJ disc due to ligament laxity and in some cases, a perforated disc. Dr. Annandale credits these diagnostic findings to practitioners that have come before him; however, until this article, there has not been a technique described to correct these problems. Drawing from his orthopedic education and experiences, he describes a procedure to access the temporomandibular joint and to correct the position of the articulating cartilage within the TMJ.

> The operation is upon the same principle as that which I have described and successfully carried out in connexion with the displacement of the semilunar cartilages of the knee-joint.

Having a strong background in knee and hip surgery, his operative technique is based upon his experiences with correcting the "semi-lunar cartilages of the knee joint." He describes the incision with anatomic landmarks, careful dissection including management of "bleeding vessels," and division of the lateral joint capsule. The disc would then be encountered and he would discuss a plication method which we continue to utilize today.

> The inter-articular cartilage was found to be loosened from its attachments, and much more movable than usual. The cartilage, having been seized with artery forceps, was drawn into position, and a catgut suture passed through it and the periosteum and other tissues at the outer margin of the joint.

Dr. Annandale's incision and dissection methods have undergone some minor adaptations over the past 135 years as surgical instrumentation and technology has advanced. However, the disc plication technique that he describes is largely unchanged on today's operating rooms.

Dr. Annandale goes on to discuss two cases where he utilized this method.

Case 1 describes a 38-year-old female who had an inciting event which progressed to a disorder where she suffered left TMJ pain and multiple close lock episodes. She underwent the procedure that he described and reported that her disc was found to be "loosened from it's attachment." After the aforementioned disc plication method, he reported "natural" joint function where she could "separate the jaws perfectly without locking or catch."

Case 2 describes an 18-year-old female who also had an inciting event and subsequently developed hypo-mobility of the left joint.

> The usual operation was performed, and the left inter-articular cartilage, being found loosened, was stitched in position with a catgut suture as in the former case. The wound was healed at the end of a week and she left the infirmary….with perfect and proper movement of the jaws.

In both of these cases, Dr. Annandale describes a clinical picture that we see quite often in our practices. In 1887, his surgical treatment is not unlike procedures we perform today. This landmark article was the beginning of a windfall of surgical publications regarding maladies and surgical management of the TMJ patient.

In 1909, Lanz discussed a discectomy procedure to help patients with painful disc displacement [2]. In 1914, Murphy discussed using the temporalis fascia with fat as a pedicled flap between the condyle and fossa in ankylosed joints [3]. In the 1940s and 1950s, the authors continued to popularize disc removal for treatment of the diseased joint with intra-articular adhesions [4, 5].

Increasing the joint space was another method to alleviate TMJ discomfort. This was achieved with a high condylar shave in 1957 by Henny. His technique served to increase the joint space via an intracapsular approach. Increasing the joint space via an extracapsular approach was achieved with the vertical ramus osteotomy technique which was popularized by Sir Terrance Ward [6, 7].

The concept of myofascial pain was first introduced in 1904 by Gowers as fibrositis and further studied in the 1950s–1980s by Travell [8, 9]. This notion brought about some skepticism with respect to surgical management of intra-articular problems. Symptoms persisted in surgical candidates, despite conservative efforts and in the 1970s, disc displacement became universally accepted as a concept and disc repair and plication became a mainstay of treatment [6].

Wilke's work on structural and functional alterations in the TMJ followed by his classification system formalized, categorized, and set treatment rationale for TMJ surgery as we know it today. His groundbreaking work in the 1970s and 1980s gave way to furthering surgical acceptance during this time [10–12].

The 1980s brought about a darker period for TMJ surgery due to difficulty with alloplastic reconstruction. Teflon-Proplast implants used as an interpositional material to replace the TMJ disc were utilized during this time and resulted in fragmentation of the material with an aggressive foreign body reaction within the patient. This product was removed from the market in 1988. Silicone "silastic" material was introduced and used in a similar fashion. This material also showed evidence of fragmentation but not as severe as the Teflon-Proplast. Silicone is no longer available for permanent implantation but can still be used as a temporary material to promote connective tissue growth and decrease adhesion formation. These materials as permanent reconstructive efforts caused significant complications for patients and alloplastic joint reconstruction was questioned [6, 13].

Despite these failures in the 1980s, the need for treatment of end stage temporomandibular joint disease remained. In 1995, using materials that were well successfully researched and utilized in orthopedic surgery, Mecuri and Wolford reported positive preliminary results using a TMJ replacement system with a patient-fitted custom CAD/CAM total TMJ replacement device, and in 2000, Quinn introduced a stock TMJ replacement system using these similar orthopedic materials. The functional aspect of these joints has a fossa consisting of an ultra-high molecular weight polyethylene, and the condylar head component is constructed with a chromium–cobalt–molybdenum alloy. These devices have proven to be highly successful over the past 2+ decades and have become the standard of care in total TMJ replacement surgery [14, 15].

Surgical management of the TMJ patient has come a long way since Dr. Annandale's description of 2 successful disc plication cases in 1887. The radiographic and clinical tools that we have today were not available at that time, yet he was able to diagnose and treat these patients successfully and we continue to use and build upon his methods today. Our surgical armamentarium now includes arthrocentesis, diagnostic arthroscopy, operative arthroscopy, arthroplasty with eminectomy, discectomy, autogenous grafting and flaps, and TMJ replacement surgery. As oral and maxillofacial surgeons, we owe our TMJ surgical successes to Dr. Annandale and many others for their diligence, innovation, successes, and failures. We will continue to carry the torch.

## Legacy

Dr. Thomas Annandale is known for many firsts. He performed the first successful orchiopexy of an undescended testicle. He also performed the first meniscus repair in a knee and was the first to excise an acoustic neuroma. He also operated on the hip, fingers, and toes and performed abdominal surgery. He was well educated, respected by his peers, and accomplished as a surgeon and academic author [16, 17].

## Early and Family Life

Thomas Annandale was born on February 2, 1838, in Newcastle upon Tyne, England. He was born to Dr. Thomas Annandale (also a surgeon) and Elizabeth Johnston. He married Mary Eveline Nelson in 1874 in Edinburgh, Scotland, and had at least 6 children [17].

## Education and Career

Dr. Annandale began his studies at Bruce's Academy in Newcastle. His interest and experience in medicine began with an apprenticeship with his father who. He continued his education at the Newcastle Infirmary followed by more formal medical and surgical training at Edinburgh University. He became a member of the Royal

College of Surgeons of England in 1859 and a fellow in 1888. He became a fellow of the Royal College of Surgeons of Edinburgh in 1863. He worked as a house surgeon at the Royal Infirmary in Edinburgh under Scottish surgeon, Dr. James Syme from 1861 to 1870. He became a fellow of the Royal Society of Edinburgh in 1867. He became Regius Professor of Clinical Surgery at the University of Edinburgh in 1877. Dr. Annandale was Surgeon-General to the Royal Company of Archers from May 1900 until his death[1818,19].

Dr. Annandale published extensively in all aspects of surgery. He won the Jacksonian prize on his dissertation of *The Malformations, Diseases, and Injuries of the Fingers and Toes and their Treatment*. He also received the gold medal at the University of Edinburgh Medical School for his theses *On the Injuries and Diseases of the Hip Joint* [18, 19].

Dr. Thomas Annandale passed suddenly on December 20, 1907, at the age of 69. He was buried at the Dean Cemetery in Western Edinburgh [18, 19] (Fig. 8.1).

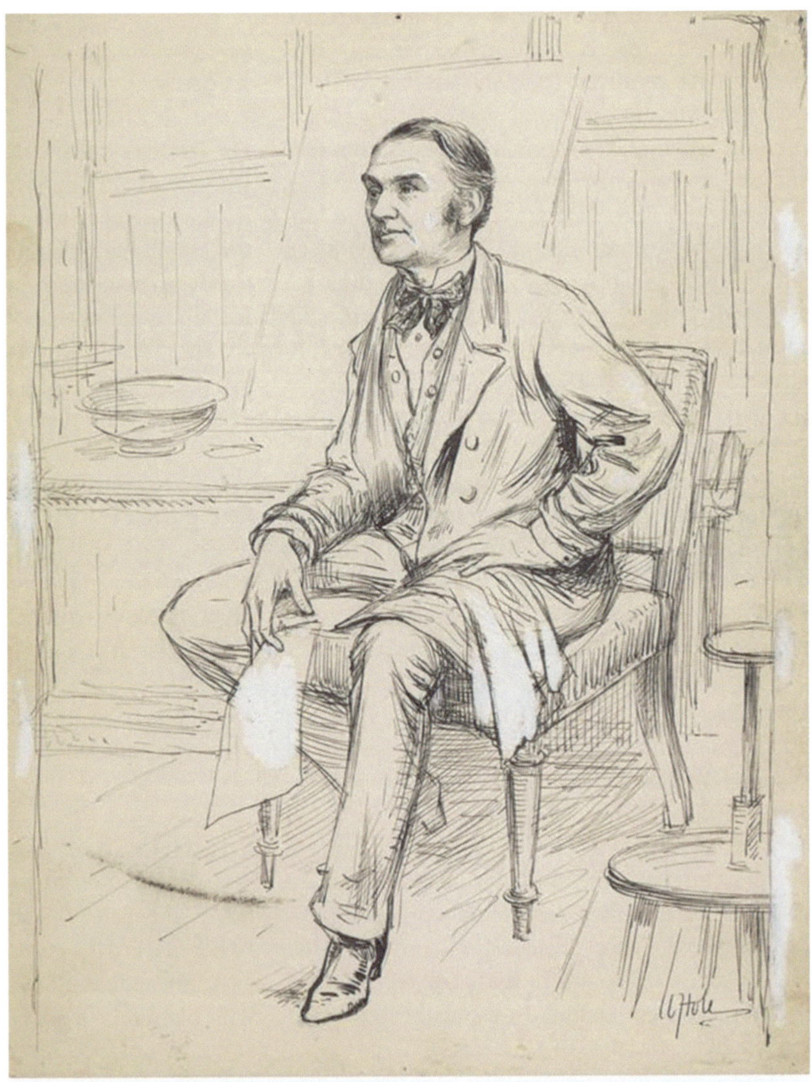

**Fig. 8.1** Professor Thomas Annandale, 1838–1907. Professor of Clinical Surgery at Edinburgh University, 1884. (Creative Commons CC by NC)

## References


1. Thomaidis V, Tsoucalas G, Fiska A. The Hippocratic method for the reduction of the mandibular dislocation, an ancient Greek procedure still in use in maxillofacial surgery. Acta Med Acad. 2018;47(1):139–43.
2. Lanz A. Discitismandibularis. Zentralbl Chir. 1909;36:289–91.
3. Murphy JB. Arthroplasty for intra-articular bony and fibrous ankylosis of temporomandibular articulation: Report of nine cases. JAMA. 1914;62(23):1783–94.
4. Boman K. Temporomandibular joint arthrosis and its treatment by extirpation of the disc. Acta Chir Scand. 1947;95(Suppl 118):1.
5. Dingman RO, Moorman WC. Meniscectomy in treatment of lesions of the temporomandibular joint. J Oral Surg. 1951;9:214.
6. Indresano AT, Mobati DA. History of temporomandibular joint surgery. Oral Maxillofac Surg Clin North Am. 2006;18(3):283–9.
7. Ward TG. Surgery of the mandibular joint. Ann R Coll Surg Engl. 1961;28(3):139–52.
8. Travell J, Rinzler SH. The myofascial genesis of pain. Postgrad Med. 1952;11(5):425–34.
9. Gowers WR. Lumbago: its lessons and analogues. Br Med J. 1904;1:117–21.
10. Wilkes CH. Structural and functional alterations of the temporomandibular joint. Northwest Dent. 1978;57:287–94.
11. Wilkes CH. Internal derangements of the temporomandibular joint. Pathological variations. Arch Otolaryngol Head Neck Surg. 1989;115:469–77.
12. Wilkes CH. Arthrography of the temporomandibular joint in patients with the TMJ pain-dysfunction syndrome. Minn Med. 1978;61:645–52.
13. DeMerle M, Nafiu OO, Aronovich S. Temporomandibular joint discectomy with abdominal fat graft versus temporalis myofascial flap: a comparative study. J Oral Maxillofac Surg. 2017;75(6):1137–43.
14. Mercuri LG, Wolford LM, Sanders B, White RD, Hurder A, Henderson W. Custom CAD/CAM total temporomandibular joint reconstruction system: preliminary multicenter report. J Oral Maxillofac Surg. 1995;53(2):106–15.
15. Mercuri LG. Temporomandibular joint replacement devices—dark past to challenging future. Stomatol Dis Sci. 2019;3:3.
16. Di Matteo B, Tarabella V, Filardo G, Viganò A, Tomba P, Marcacci M. Thomas Annandale: the first meniscus repair. Knee Surg Sports Traumatol Arthrosc. 2013;21(9):1963–6.
17. "Regius Chair of Clinical Surgery" (PDF). Edinburgh University. Archived from the original (PDF) on 11 July 2012.
18. Stephen L. Annandale, Thomas. In: Dictionary of National Biography, vol. 1. London: Smith, Elder; 1885.
19. Bryan BA. Annandale, Thomas. In: Oxford Dictionary of National Biography (online ed.). Oxford: Oxford University Press.

# Part II

# World War I Pioneers

# Sir Harold Delf Gillies: A New Principle in the Treatment of Congenital Cleft Palate and Its Mechanical Counterpart. British Medical Journal. Vol 1, No 3140, pp. 335–338. March 5 1921

9

Matthew Stephens, Daniel M. Roistacher, and Michael D. Turner

**Abstract**

Sir Harold Delf Gillies (1882–1960) was a New Zealand surgeon whose practices greatly influenced the advancement of modern maxillofacial and plastic surgery. The first part of this chapter will describe and put into context Gillies' novel surgical technique to correct congenital cleft palate, which he developed as part of a combined prosthetic treatment with his colleague W. Kelsey Fry. Originally published in 1921 in the *British Medical Journal*, this method provided improved mastication, soft palate function, and limited damage to developing dentition when compared to other contemporaneous technique. The second part of this chapter will review key points of Gillies' life including his early childhood and education, formative experience treating facial injuries sustained on the battlefields of World War I, innovations in reconstructive plastic surgery, as well as his later career and legacy.

**Keywords**

Harold Gillies · Kelsey Fry · Sidcup · Cleft palate · Maxillofacial injuries · Plastic surgery

## The Gillies and Fry Cleft Palate Repair

The surgical treatment of congenital cleft lip and palate has experienced considerable innovation over time. In history, primary lip repairs were documented as early as the fifth century AD in China; however, the repair of the soft palate has only been described in recent centuries. Prior to the introduction of general anesthesia, such repairs were often not possible to complete, and years passed before the more comprehensive procedures were feasibly attempted. The experience gained by surgeons treating battlefield injuries of the First World War served to influence the development of new plastic and maxillofacial surgical techniques including the management of the cleft lip and palate. Two of these surgeons were Harold D. Gillies of Queen's Hospital, Sidcup, and W. Kelsey Fry of Guy's Hospital, who together published the first recommendation for a delayed

M. Stephens
Private Practice, San Francisco, CA, USA
e-mail: matthew.stephens@mountsinai.org

D. M. Roistacher · M. D. Turner (✉)
Division of Oral and Maxillofacial Surgery, Icahn School of Medicine at Mount Sinai, New York, NY, USA
e-mail: daniel.roistacher@einsteinmed.edu; daniel.roistacher@mountsinai.org; Michael.turner@mountsinai.org


S. R. Aziz, M. D. Turner (eds.), *Classic Papers and Pioneers in Maxillofacial and Oral Surgery*,
https://doi.org/10.1007/978-3-031-63246-4_9

closure of the hard palate: "A New Principle in the Surgical Treatment of 'Congenital Cleft Palate,' and its Mechanical Counterpart. The British Medical Journal. Volume 1, Issue 3140. March 1921."

In this seminal work, Gillies and Fry explained their ideal goals for the treatment of patients with cleft lip and palate and opined on the deficiencies of current outcomes:

> The ideals to be aimed at are: Perfect speech; perfect mastication; normal nasal respiratory function; and, in so far as a displaced maxilla causes deformity, a normal bony contour. The success of a palate operation is often gauged merely by the completeness of the surgical closure. This should not be so, as it is hoped to show that successful closure of a wide cleft by any of the present-day operations is incompatible with the full attainment of the above ideals.

Although there were many contemporaneous methods in use, the "present-day operations" Gillies and Fry referred to were the techniques by Brophy, Lane, and von Langenbeck. Truman Brophy in 1901 described the use of metal wires passed transversely across the maxilla to draw a cleft defect together in patients younger than 3 months of age. This technique resulted in a narrowed maxilla and destruction of permanent tooth buds. Although Brophy would disagree, Gillies and Fry stated that these outcomes occurred far too often. Another method was developed by Sir William Arbuthnot Lane who closed palatal defects with periosteum and mucous membrane. This technique, on average, led to a rigid scarred soft palate that was forwardly displaced and provided insufficient velopharyngeal closure. Bernard von Langenbeck, in 1861, described the placement of incisions along the oral side of the cleft and laterally along the posterior alveolar ridge to raise two separate mucoperiosteal flaps that are brought medially to close the defect. This technique and its modifications are still often used today for repair of isolated cleft palates. The Langenbeck approximation led to good closure of the hard palate and adequate mobility of the soft palate; however, in wide defects, the result was of a palate that was too short. Malocclusion was a consequence of all three of these techniques, particularly when the hard palate was repaired at an early age, as in the Lane and Langenbeck procedures. Narrowing of the nasal passages and poor facial appearance were other outcomes that Gillies and Fry described.

Gillies and Fry sought to eliminate these results by a two part treatment using both surgical and prosthetic intervention. The surgical technique involved the detachment of the soft palate from the hard palate and suturing the two halves of the soft palate together along a prepared raw surface on their medial aspects. The outcome of this operation was a lengthened soft palate situated further posterior in the pharynx. This however resulted in a larger hard palate defect. To address this and decrease the risk of the soft palate forming an anteriorly displaced scar contracture, Gillies recommended the use of either a small mucoperiosteal palate flap or a skin overlay graft. He believed that these would cover and protect the raw anterior edge of the soft palate.

The hard palate defect itself was to be obturated prosthetically. Fry described the benefits of this combined treatment as an easier prosthetic closure of the hard palate and reduced deviation of the dental arch and improved facial appearance. The role of a dental prosthesis is as follows: to aid in feeding by preventing food entering nasal cavity, to hold the epithelial flap or onlay in proper position postoperatively, to maintain repaired position of soft palate by preventing it being drawn forward by scar tissue, and to restore the hard palate defect. Postoperatively, if additional intervention was necessary to obtain adequate soft palate contact with the pharynx, Fry recommended an appliance be fabricated to gradually stretch the soft palate to a proper position. A permanent appliance for obturation of the hard palate defect was made of hard rubber, with or without gold. If obturation of the anterior soft palate was necessary, a softer "velum rubber" was used. All the prostheses were ideally fabricated preoperatively so that they would be available for use and could be adjusted.

This combined surgical and prosthetic approach, while a remarkable innovation, was not the first use of a mechanical device for the

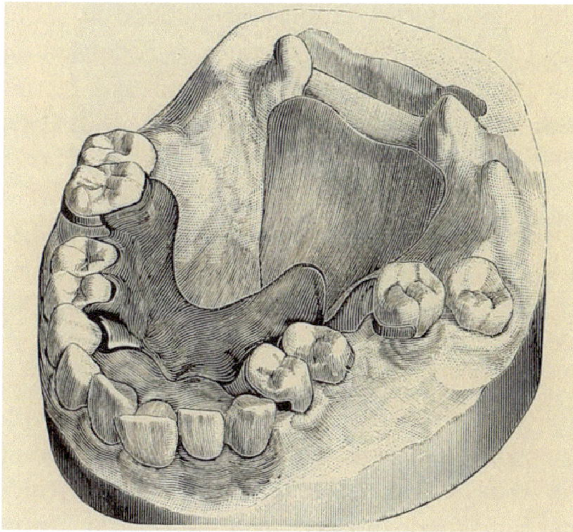

**Fig. 9.1** Dr. Norman Kingsley's Artificial Velum. (Adapted from 'A Manual of the Injuries and Surgical Diseases of the Face, Mouth, and Jaws' by John Sayre Marshall, published 1897, via public domain)

treatment of cleft palates. One notable advancement was described by Dr. Norman W. Kinglsey (Fig. 9.1). In the mid-nineteenth century, Dr. Kingsley, using Charles Goodyear's vulcanized rubber, was able to improve the appliances so that they were both accurate and adjustable. Another benefit of the Kinglsey device was that it had good retention and moved well in conjunction with the soft palate muscles which resulted in a decrease in food regurgitation and improved speech. These earlier techniques, such as this one, paved the way for the later Gillies and Fry method. Per Fry, "It is enough to say that this combined treatment promises to solve the treatment of these most difficult cases, both from the surgical and the dental aspect."

## Early Life: University and Early Career

Harold Delf Gillies was born on June 17, 1882, in Dunedin in the Otago Province of New Zealand. Gillies' family origins are in the Isle of Bute. His grandfather uprooted the family and moved them to New Zealand when he became a magistrate in Dunedin. Gillies was the youngest of eight children born to Robert Gillies and Emily Street. After his father's sudden death from a coronary aneurysm in 1886, Gillies and his family relocated to Auckland. It was here Gillies began his formal studies at Wanganui Collegiate School. By 1901, Gillies' educational pursuits brought him to Cambridge, England, where he had been granted a chapel scholarship and attended Gonville and Caius College to study medicine.

Aside from his academic excellence, Gillies also had prodigious athletic prowess. As a young man at Wanganui College, he captained the school's first cricket eleven and was considered by some to be one of the best young players in New Zealand. Gillies won a rowing blue while at Cambridge and rowed number 7 for Cambridge in the 1904 Boat Race. Gillies also had become one of the premier amateur golfers in England. He represented England three-times against Scotland and was a plus-2 handicap on the greens. Gillies even made it as far as the fifth round of the British Amateur Golf tournament.

In 1906 at the age of 24, Gillies qualified to finish his training at St. Bartholomew's Hospital in London. Gillies' surgical precocity endeared him to his colleagues. George E. Gask, an Assistant Surgeon at Barts remarked that "[Gillies] was the best house surgeon we have had at St. Bartholomew's for some years." Gillies finished his medical training at St. Bartholomew's Hospital in 1908, and shortly thereafter, became a fellow of the Royal College of Surgeons in 1910. At Bart's, Gillies developed an interest in otolaryngology. He soon became chief assistant to the Registrar at the Hospital for Diseases of the Throat in Golden Square, the premier laryngology hospital in England.

Despite having already established a reputation as an academician, Gillies found the lure of private practice irresistible and applied to be private assistant to Sir Milsom Rees. Sir Milsom was the laryngologist to the King and Queen and a consultant to the Royal Opera house and was considered to be one of the best laryngologists in London. The story of Gillies' interview with Sir

Milsom was quite unusual. When Gillies showed up to meet Rees on Harley Street, having spent a considerable sum on dress for the occasion, Sir Milsom barely regarded his academic accomplishments or his professional experience but instead, Rees took great curiosity in his exploits on the golf course. At one point during the infamous interview, Sir Milsom even presented his golf clubs for an exasperated Gillies to inspect. As the story goes, Rees offered Gillies the position seemingly as an afterthought while on his way out the door to see a consult. Regardless, Gillies' surgical practice flourished. His partnership with Rees lasted until World War I broke out and Gillies' career took on a different trajectory.

## World War I

In 1915, Gillies volunteered with the Red Cross and was stationed in Hoogstad. France. It was here he met French-American dentist, Auguste Valadier, who had established a successful unit for treating jaw injuries at Wimereux. Gillies filled a convenient role for Valadier, as the latter was not credentialed to operate without the supervision of a medical doctor. Working with Valadier, Gillies became interested in facial reconstruction. This was further catalyzed when he visited and observed the surgeon Hippolyte Morestin at Val de Grace Hospital. Morestin was a talented Creole surgeon who had found great success in using adipose and cartilaginous grafts for the repair of extensive facial lesions. After witnessing Morestin operate and the results he obtained, Gillies wrote:

> I stood spell bound as he removed half of a face distorted with a horrible cancer and then deftly turned a neck flap to restore not only the cheek but the side of the nose and lip in one shot... at the time it was the most thrilling thing I had ever seen. I fell in love with the work on the spot.

Gillies returned to Britain and in 1916 convinced Army Surgeon-General Alfred Keogh to establish a unit devoted to the treatment of maxillofacial injuries. Gillies was allotted wards at the Cambridge Military Hospital at Aldershot. In its beginning, Gillies had to find and recruit patients to be treated at his unit. Famously, Gillies bought 10£-worth of baggage tags addressed to himself at Aldershot. The tags were given to the War Office with instructions to distribute to soldiers who had suffered facial injuries. Patients began to trickle into Aldershot in the days and weeks following. Then, all at once, the casualties poured in. After the first day of the Battle of the Somme, some 2000 soldiers with facial wounds arrived at Aldershot over a period of 10 days. Gillies found no trouble in convincing Sir Arbuthnot Lane, then the Head of Army Surgery, that the Aldershot's facilities were inadequate for the volume of facial casualties they were treating.

The government secured a disused Jacobean mansion on the border of Sidcup, Kent, to build what would become a facility devoted entirely to the treatment of facial injuries. The Queen's Hospital, as it famously became known, was constructed as a series of convalescing wards with a 1000-bed capacity. Within these walls, Gillies assembled a multidisciplinary team of doctors, dentists, anesthetists, technicians, and artists to treat complex facial injuries (Fig. 9.2). Gillies was among the first to employ painters, sculptors, and photographers to meticulously document his work. Henry Tonks, also a surgeon, was one of the artists whose watercolors and drawings helped to document the discoveries made at Sidcup. His detailed drawings were included in many of Gillies' ensuing publications.

One other important member of the team at The Queen's Hospital was dental surgeon and collaborator, Kelsey Fry. Gillies and Fry had worked together at Aldershot prior to Sidcup. Gillies made use of Fry's expertise in oral surgery and prosthodontics skills in his multidisciplinary approach to patient care. Fry became the director of a large team of dentists and dental technicians who designed the prostheses that helped restore masticatory function for soldiers

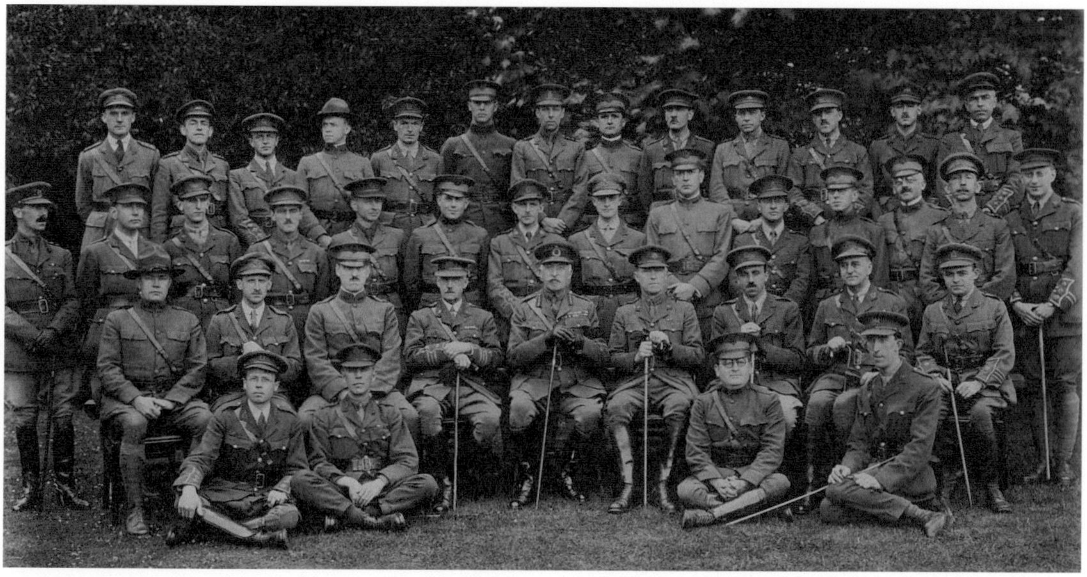

**Fig. 9.2** Staff of the Queen's Hospital, Sidcup, during a visit by H.R.H. The Duke of Connaught, June 4, 1918. Harold Gillies seated second row, third from right. (Adapted from photo by Sydney S. Walbridge, License CC BY 2.0, via Archives New Zealand)

with jaw injuries. Fry is also credited with helping Ivan Magill and Stanley Rowbotham pioneer endotracheal intubation. In fact, the first nasoendotracheal tube was said to have been designed and created in Kelsey Fry's dental lab.

The Queen's hospital became an incubator for innovation in facial reconstruction. Led by Gillies, the technical challenges faced at Sidcup accelerated the advancement in surgical technique. Gillies recognized that the post-operative outcomes when just using local flaps and direct closure of the injuries were inadequate and that tissue had to be imported from elsewhere. Gillies and his team developed advanced tissue transfer techniques that are still in use today. Examples of these techniques are the tubed pedicle flap, the temporalis transfer flap, and a variety of others (Fig. 9.3).

Other lessons learned from Sidcup included the lining of flaps, the importance of treating underlying infection, and the general restoration of form and function using both artificial and non-artificial materials. Gillies and his team treated over 5000 patients at Sidcup and performed over 11,000 procedures. Gillies' appointment ended in 1919 and slowly, the pioneering work done at the Queen's Hospital was transferred over to its spiritual successor, The Queen Mary's Hospital in Roehampton in 1923.

Gillies' observations and surgical innovations from the war were published in 1920 in his first textbook, *Plastic Surgery of the Face*.

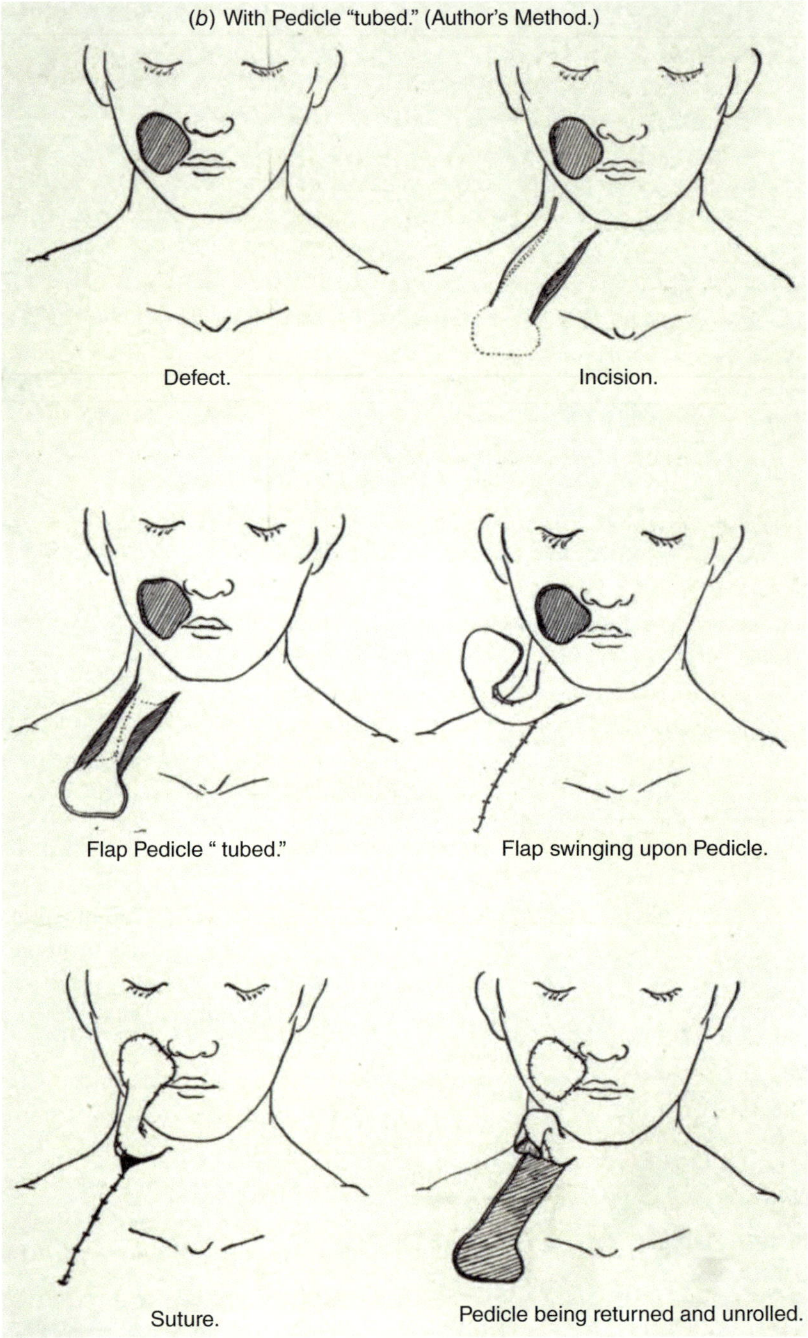


**Fig. 9.3** Technique for the Tubed Pedicle Flap from Harold Gillies' Plastic Surgery of the Face, public domain, from University of Toronto via Internet Archive

## Post-World War I Career

Though his accomplishments after leaving Sidcup were dwarfed by his achievements made during World War I, Gillies continued to push the boundaries of possibilities in facial surgery. In lieu of returning to a lucrative career as a private practice laryngologist, Gillies elected to stay in the fledgling field of plastic surgery. Gillies took a position at his old hospital, St. Bartholomew's, but also began a private practice in order to pay his bills. Gillies spent this time refining his techniques for rhinoplasties and breast reconstruction. Over time, his practice grew in size and became increasingly busy. Despite this, he continued to publish in *The Lancet* and other prestigious medical journals. In 1930, Gillies was knighted by King George V. His friend and collaborator, Kelsey Fry was also honored with a CBE in 1951.

At the dawn of World War II, Gillies became an honorary brigadier with RAMC. He was deployed to Rooksdown House, as part of the Park Prewitt Mental Hospital near Basingstoke, where he established another maxillofacial unit. His expertise was invaluable because of the amount and extent of facial wounds that were treated.

After World War II, Gillies remained in Basingstoke to operate at Roehampton. In 1957, he published his second textbook titled *The Principles and Art of Plastic Surgery,* which he co-authored with Ralph Millard. This expanded on the fundamentals established in *Plastic Surgery of the Face*.

## The Legacy

The influence Gillies had on modern surgical practice and plastic surgery cannot be understated.

> Gillies invented plastic surgery. There was no plastic surgery before he came. Everything since then no matter whose name be attached to it was started by Gillies—Sir William Heneage Ogilvie

Gillies helped to establish the British Association of Plastic Surgeons and in 1947 was elected the foundation's first president. Among Gillies' other accolades are honorary fellow of the American College of Surgeons, The Royal Society of Medicine, London, and honorary president of the International Society of Plastic Surgeons.

Gillies' advances in surgical technique were revolutionary, but his greatest contribution may have been in shaping the careers of other pioneers in facial surgery of the era. Gillies' first cousin, Archibald McIndoe, came to England in 1930, to find work as a general surgeon. McIndoe became inspired by the works of his cousin and soon became an accomplished plastic surgeon himself. Tommy Kilner, who was at Sidcup, and Rainsford Mowlem were also mentored by Gillies. Together, Gillies, McIndoe, Kilner, and Mowlem made up "the big four" of plastic surgery in the mid-twentieth century and were responsible for nursing the specialty during its infant phase.

Gillies skill as a surgeon can be summarized as meticulous. As Cecil Hogg recalled, GIllies was rumored to "spend an hour putting in an accurate suture line only to decide that it was not good enough, and then to take them all out and start again." Many of Gillies' aphorisms such as "never throw away anything until you are sure you will not need it" and "never do today what can honorably be put off until tomorrow" are now regarded as essential credo in facial surgery.

To his patients, Gillies was known for his professional and sensitive demeanor. Another side to Gillies, well known to his friends and colleagues, was his wry sense of humor and often mischievous antics. Golf was one such outlet for Gillies' whimsical nature. Gillies was known for teeing off of beer bottles, or switching out his playing-partner's balls for eggs. He once removed his coat and trousers at a dinner party to humorously demonstrate the utility of a specialized coat hanger he had designed. Gillies was known to don elaborate disguises in order to entertain his patients and kept an extensive wardrobe of false beards and costumes. On Gillies' waggish nature, Ralph Millard remarked, "Such genius deserves a touch of leniency, for ascension to such bewildering heights may require occasional compensatory descents into juvenile delinquency."

Gillies passed away in 1960 at the age of 78 from presumed complications of long-standing arterial disease. The legacy he left behind can be considered no less than a watershed moment in maxillofacial surgery.

# The Evolution of Oral Surgery: President's Address. Journal of the Royal Society of Medicine. Section of Odontology. Vol. 44, pp. 139–143. February 1951

10

Abrar Shamim and Shahid R. Aziz

**Abstract**

Wartime injuries to the maxillofacial complex during WWI provided the basis for advancements in both maxillofacial and plastic surgery. Sir William Kelsey Fry served in many capacities to the British armed forces; however, his role in the treatment of traumatic fractures was most critical in that the specialty of oral and maxillofacial surgery was born and recognized in Europe, although across the Atlantic the Americans had already done so through the likes of Simon Hullihen and James Garretson. Sir William's 1951 Presidential Address "The Evolution of Oral Surgery" is discussed and his accomplishments relating to oral and maxillofacial surgery presented in the context of WWI and II.

**Keywords**

Maxillofacial surgery · Sir William Kelsey Fry · Trauma surgery · World War

A. Shamim
Department of Oral and Maxillofacial Surgery, Harvard School of Dental Medicine, Boston, MA, USA
e-mail: ashamim@mgh.harvard.edu

S. R. Aziz (✉)
Division of Oral and Maxillofacial Surgery, Department of Otolaryngology, Hackensack Meridian School of Medicine, Nutley, NJ, USA
e-mail: azizsr@sdm.rutgers.edu; Shahid.aziz@hmhn.org

Sir William Kelsey Fry, born on March 18, 1899, is regarded as a visionary and founder of the field of maxillofacial surgery, permitted by his broad dual training in medicine and dentistry, authorship of one of the original textbooks on maxillofacial trauma, and service in the British armed forces during WWI and II. He studied at Hurstpierpoint and Guy's Hospital, obtaining qualifications in MRCS (Membership of the Royal College of Surgeons of Great Britain and Ireland) and LRCP (Licentiate of the Royal College of Physicians) in 1912 and LDS RCS (Licensee in Dental Surgery by the Royal College of Surgeons) in 1913. He also obtained by election the titles of FDS (Faculty of Dental Surgery) in 1947 and FRCS (Fellow of the Royal College of Surgeons) in 1952.

In the pre-WWI era, treatment of diseases and injuries of the jaws was directly in the scope of practice of neither surgery nor dentistry. Rather, an awkward interplay between them prevailed, fueled by lack of training in dental rehabilitation by surgeons and lack of training in sound surgical principles by dentists, alongside the lack of textbooks that adequately tied these fields together. Sir William Fry's wartime experience in the treatment of injuries of the head and face, which were the most vulnerable during trench warfare, provided a basis for the scope and need of maxillofacial surgery as a specialty; it was borne in parallel with plastic surgery through Kelsey Fry's collaborative work alongside Harold Gillies, who


S. R. Aziz, M. D. Turner (eds.), *Classic Papers and Pioneers in Maxillofacial and Oral Surgery*, https://doi.org/10.1007/978-3-031-63246-4_10

achieved great strides in the practice of plastic surgery. The accomplishments in maxillofacial surgery were also shared by Sir Auguste Charles Valadier, although this chapter will focus on Fry's contributions.

Sir William's positioned himself as an oral surgeon during a time where the organizing demarcation between the practice of general surgery and the rising specialty of oral surgery was indistinct, and many aspects of modern-day oral surgery were introduced and practiced by general surgeons. Fry wrote, "although the history of oral surgery is closely intermingled with that of dentistry, most of the advances have come through surgeons rather than dentists" [1]. Sir William noted his observations of surgeons Sir Charters Symonds and Sir Arbuthnot Lane who participated in the extraction of third molars and repair of facial clefts. Although in the current day such cases are often encompassed by the specialty fields of stomatology and oral surgery, it became apparent to Sir William that conditions of the jaw, including injuries, diseases, and malformations "belonged to a no-man's land" during the earlier half of the twentieth century. Therefore, he took it upon himself to use his experiences in the early development of the specialty to demonstrate how an intersection of surgery and dentistry is paramount to improving treatment of diseases in the head and neck.

Sir William Fry in his 1951 President's Address "The Evolution of Oral Surgery" addressed the scope and boundaries of the developing specialty and its bridging function between surgery and dentistry [1]. The jurisdiction of jaw fractures was not only unclear but also neglected. Although general surgeons treated fractures of the jaws in Europe at that time, textbooks on general surgery failed to cover jaw appropriately, and neither did orthopedic textbooks. Sir William realized that the Americans on the other side of the Atlantic had textbooks covering jaw fractures, and these originated from pioneers in the field of dentistry. It also seemed odd to him that during surgical resection of jaw tumors (adamantinomas) that no reconstructive effort of the excised site was made, leaving the patient with a debilitating void, albeit in the absence of active tumors. He described that if a dentist were only present during such surgical procedures, collaboration with the surgeon would massively improve the functional outcomes:

> I have met many examples where a surgeon operating alone has produced a condition which, although resulting in a cure, might have been considerably improved from the point of view of the comfort and the functional ability of the patient, had the dental surgeon been called into consultation with the surgeon at the time of operation

As a solution to this problem, he takes the position that one provider may be adequately trained to combine these services in the form of oral surgery, pushing back on those who suggested that such a broad training becomes too extensive for one man to endeavor. Fry mentions the following, based on his own training, which has undoubtedly influenced the training of oral and maxillofacial surgeons worldwide to date:

> a new type [of dental trainee] arose: one who, although he fully appreciated the value of technique, also saw the need for a fuller knowledge of general medicine and surgery… [however] the oral surgeon whose hands are unaccustomed to the bench is of little use. How can one treat a difficult [jaw] fracture without knowing how to construct a splint? Or prepare the mouth for a complete denture without knowing the exact type of restoration that is to be inserted?

Sir William explained how a proper oral surgeon could be trained with instruction in both surgery and dental rehabilitation. The issue, as he described, was that there was simply insufficient overlap in the education of general surgeons with technical prosthetic skills learned by dentists, while there was insufficient training in sound surgical principles in dental training. This begged the question of whether an oral surgeon should be trained initially in surgery through medicine and then in dental technique or vice versa, to which Fry writes:

> The oral surgeon must have a more than average knowledge of prosthetic technique: knowledge which takes years of application to acquire. At the same time I am sure that a man who has a general medical training, but who has had little general surgical experience, can acquire his technique during his training in oral surgery, provided that he is constantly in contact with the general surgeons.

He goes on to describe house appointments, registrarships, and rotations within both general and specialized hospitals that he believed to be necessary for adequate surgical training of a dentist. Sir William had a unique perspective of the fusion of these two fields and how it may be achieved as a result of the collaborative relationship he developed with ENT surgeon Harold Gillies after the First Great War in treating injuries of the maxillofacial complex.

## Sir William Kelsey Fry's Life: Pre-WWI to Post-WWII

Soon after completing his education in 1913, Sir Kelsey Fry was commissioned to join the Royal Welch Fusiliers as Medical Officer. This was a time where dentists were not enlisted for their professional services but rather enlisted as combatants unless they had medical training. Those who joined and led specialty surgical teams to treat injuries of the jaws and face established many principles of modern-day oral and maxillofacial surgery. Kelsey Fry's dual training in medicine and dentistry facilitated his enlistment as Medical Officer; however, he maintained years later that it was in fact his comfort in riding horse-back that led him to his enlistment in the Royal Army Medical Corps (RAMC) rather than his accomplishments in medicine [2].

Sir William served in both Great Wars, as Medical Officer in the RAMC during WWI and consultant to the Royal Air Force and Emergency Medical Service during WWII. The role of medical officer came with many perils and required bravery: to retrieve injured soldiers from the field and manage wards with severely mutilated combat men. He was injured in battle on two separate occasions, one during the 1915 Battle of Festubert in which he was shot in the back of both legs while retrieving injured soldiers, for which he received the Military Cross for bravery on May 9, 1915. He returned to the field but was injured again on August 29, 1916, when his medical post was hit by shelling [3].

After his second injury, in 1916 Sir William was posted to the Cambridge Hospital in Aldershot (a town in Hampshire, England), where he, alongside ENT surgeon Harold Gillies, established the first plastic and maxillofacial unit in the British army [4]. After the 1616 Battle of Somme, over 2000 soldiers with maxillofacial injuries were reported, upon which a new unit was established in 1917 by Gillies and Fry in Sidcup, in the south-east London county of Kent [5]. In this hospital, 20 or more soldiers with jaw fractures were admitted every day, and efficient treatment of these injuries led to the basis in which Fry worked alongside Harold Gillies, one of the few plastic surgeons in the country. This partnership with Gillies guided Fry's perspectives on the interrelationship of surgery and dentistry; they reconstructed the jaws and faces of 11,572 patients between Aldershot and Sidcup during the Great War [6]. He is quoted as saying to Gillies, "I'll take the hard tissues, you take the soft," although their roles often overlapped and each learned from the other's expertise. The hospital in which Kelsey Fry and Gillies established their legendary collaboration persists today as Queen Mary's Hospital, Sidcup, with a persisting oral and maxillofacial surgery service. The discipline today known as "plastic surgery" was largely pioneered by Gillies in this unit, with Sir William Kelsey Fry as his partner [7].

Sir William also played a role in the invention of the first endotracheal anesthesia tubes, which were crafted in his prosthetic dental workshop, for fellow surgeon Harold Gillies and anesthesiologists Ivan Magill and Stanley Rowbotham [4]. Ivan Magill is credited with many advances in intratracheal anesthesia during the 1920s while working at the Queen's Hospital for Facial and Jaw Injuries in Sidcup, alongside Gillies. Some of these contributions include the angulated Magill forceps used for nasotracheal intubation, various tubes, and Magill laryngoscope blade [8]. Although Sir Kelsey Fry's involvement often goes unmentioned, his expertise in prosthetics work allowed for these new devices to be manufactured and which to this day remain a critical aspect of facial surgery and has become a standard in many settings. The first Magill tubes allowed for endotracheal intubation, which was an important advancement from facemasks and other obstructive equipment, which were a problem for surgery involving the face and jaws.

After the First Great War was over and his time at the hospital in Sidcup terminated, Sir William returned to civilian life to work and teach as Assistant Dental Surgeon and Director of the Prosthetic Laboratory at Guy's Hospital in London, where he had trained prior to the war [2].

With his experience from the Great War and subsequent clinical practice, Sir William, along with colleagues, wrote a report outlining the management of jaw and facial injuries "The Treatment of Maxillo-facial injuries" (1942), which was used as a guide during the 1940s for maxillofacial injury units who lacked surgeons to treat WWII combat injuries and to educate novice surgeons who were not experienced fixing fractured jaws. Many new maxillofacial units were established during the Second Great War, with this text being used as a reference by many. During the Second Great War, Sir William's role was Consultant for the whole Dental Section of the Emergency Medical Service and Consultant to the Royal Air force [2]. This consultancy position allowed him to establish nine maxillofacial injury units throughout the country, including one at East Grinstead where he operated and taught [7, 9].

Advancements in maxillofacial surgery were abundant during his time at East Grinstead. Kelsey Fry led the development of a novel locking plate method of fracture fixation (Fig. 10.1);

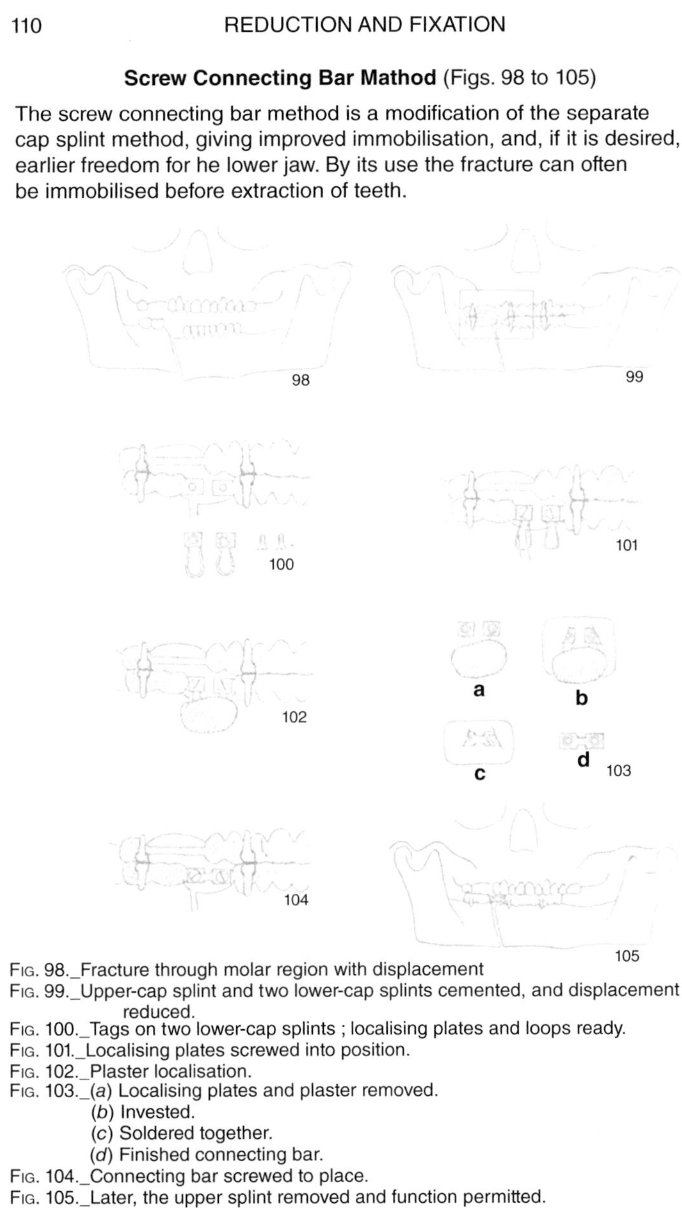

110 REDUCTION AND FIXATION

**Screw Connecting Bar Mathod** (Figs. 98 to 105)

The screw connecting bar method is a modification of the separate cap splint method, giving improved immobilisation, and, if it is desired, earlier freedom for he lower jaw. By its use the fracture can often be immobilised before extraction of teeth.



FIG. 98._Fracture through molar region with displacement
FIG. 99._Upper-cap splint and two lower-cap splints cemented, and displacement reduced.
FIG. 100._Tags on two lower-cap splints ; localising plates and loops ready.
FIG. 101._Localising plates screwed into position.
FIG. 102._Plaster localisation.
FIG. 103._(*a*) Localising plates and plaster removed.
(*b*) Invested.
(*c*) Soldered together.
(*d*) Finished connecting bar.
FIG. 104._Connecting bar screwed to place.
FIG. 105._Later, the upper splint removed and function permitted.

**Fig. 10.1** From "The Dental Treatment of Maxillofacial Injuries" (1942), page 110 [12]. Drawings of the locking plate method of mandibular fracture fixation; individual splints would be made for teeth on both fractured segments, in addition to an upper splint. The final splint position following appropriate reduction was recorded, and then a connecting bar soldered between them in a laboratory

sectional splints were positioned onto fractured segments of the jaw after appropriate reduction, upon which their final position recorded via plaster localization. They would then be removed and connected via a soldered bar in a dental lab. This technique created continuity of the jaw [10]. Throughout the procedure, the fractured jaw would be held in place to a separate splint on the intact maxilla via inter-maxillary wires to maintain the occlusion. Prior to this, during WWI, the method used for fixation in tooth-bearing patients entailed a form of model surgery, in which a model would be created and fractured. Then, a splint would be created to rearticulate the segments and then cemented onto the patient; however, this was not ideal and often done with significant difficulty [11].

## Awards and Distinctions

Sir William was awarded the 1916–1920 Cartwright Medal by the Royal College of Surgeons, awarded once every 5 years, for his essay "Treatment of Injuries of the Jaws," which was a step forward in the country's acknowledgement of both plastic surgery (which was viewed suspiciously by senior surgeons) and eventually maxillofacial surgery as specialties [13]. Sir William was awarded an honorary Doctor of Science by the McGill Faculty of Dentistry in Canada in 1955; at a special convocation to mark the 50th anniversary of the institution, Sir William gave a speech on the importance of integrating aspects of medical education into the dental education of a student, such that "he has been trained to observe for himself and to reason from his observations," as were medical doctors. His speech was described as having a "prophetic" impact on the institution [14]. He served as Dean of the Faculty of Dental Surgery at the Royal College of Surgeons from 1950 to 1953 [15] and was lecturer of oral surgery positions at the Eastman Dental Hospital (which he largely helped establish).

## Sir Kelsey Fry: The Mentor and Teacher

Serving in the war strongly influenced Sir William's career trajectory as an instructor and professor. He achieved such that his reputation as a clinical teacher brought surgeons and students around the world to learn, including American oral surgeons who had established the specialty faster than in the UK. He wrote of the following personal experience, when one soldier died after he failed to give proper instruction to other Medical Officers:

> Now that was a terrible thing to me-that I had failed to give instructions to my other officers that this man should not be put on his back, although mentally I knew what I was doing, with the result that he was put on a stretcher, and having got a fracture through both angles, he suffocated and died. I well remember wrapping him in a blanket and burying him that night, and I made up my mind that if I had an opportunity of teaching that lesson to others, I would do it. That was one of the milestones of my life.

Sir William served as clinical professor at Guy's Hospital while also opening a private practice on St. Thomas Street in London in the period after WWI. After WWII, he continued his teaching at the East Grinstead maxillofacial unit alongside Gillies and Archibald McIndoe (another pioneer in plastic surgery) and wrote essays and books to support learning of oral surgeons and others. He formed teams of dental surgeons who would provide short courses on the treatment of maxilla-facial injuries. Queen Victoria Hospital stands today where Kelsey Fry led the Grinstead maxillofacial unit during WWII and houses a busy maxillofacial surgery service today; they still treat war injuries, including those sustained by British soldiers in the War in Afghanistan.

Kelsey Fry maintained a prominent role in the management of conditions of the jaws following his wartime developments in maxillofacial surgery. In his private practice located on St. Thomas's Street in London, it was known that a jaw could not be broken within a radius of 50 miles from the city without his consultation [2]. However, Fry stressed that it was not his ambition to create a "monopoly" on such injuries: he wished to guide others to treat what he could, which he embodied in essays and texts he authored.

In 1948, Sir William was awarded the Commander of the Order of the British Empire (CBE), the highest-ranking order of the British Empire, only less than knighthood or damehood. Sir William then obtained knighthood in 1951 due to his contributions to the fields of maxillofacial and plastic surgery and the British Armed Forces during the Great Wars. He retired at the age of 70 in 1959 and moved to Bexhill, where he died on October 26, 1963, leaving behind his wife Ruby Hannah and his son Ian, who trained in medicine to become a radiologist [15]. He was remembered by his colleagues and subordinates alike as a man with a happy temperament and undying sense of humor in the hardest of times. His memory and contributions are held in many museums in the UK, including the Museum of Military Medicine, Royal College of Surgeons of England Hunterian Museum archives and collections, and Friends of the Aldershot military Museum.

We end this chapter with his prodigious words:

> God gave you ears, eyes, and hands; use them on the patient in that order."—Sir William Kelsey Fry (1899–1963)

## References


1. Fry WK. The evolution of Oral surgery: President's address. Proc R Soc Med. 1951;44:139–43. https://doi.org/10.1177/003591575104400208.
2. Great Teachers of Surgery in the Past. Sir William Kelsey Fry (1889-1963). Br J Surg. 1966;53:317–20.
3. Mayhew ER. Wounded: a new history of the Western front in world war I. Oxford: Oxford University Press; 2013; ISBN 978-0-19-932245-9.
4. Bodley P. Development of anaesthesia for plastic surgery. J R Soc Med. 1978;71:839–43. https://doi.org/10.1177/014107687807101114.
5. Stathopoulos P. Maxillofacial surgery: the impact of the great war on both sides of the trenches. Oral Maxillofac Surg. 2018;22:21. https://doi.org/10.1007/s10006-017-0659-5.
6. Friends of the Aldershot Military Museum—Garrison Herald Articles—015. https://www.friendsofthealdershotmilitarymuseum.org.uk/garrison.015.html. Accessed 11 Jun 2022.
7. Meikle MC. The evolution of plastic and maxillofacial surgery in the twentieth century: the Dunedin connection. Surgeon. 2006;4:325–34. https://doi.org/10.1016/S1479-666X(06)80010-7.
8. APPLIANCES AND PREPARATIONS. Br Med J. 1920;2:670.
9. DeLyzer T. What's in a nose: the changing face of plastic surgery. 2008. https://doi.org/10.11575/PRISM/10353.
10. Rowe NL. The history of the treatment of Maxillofacial trauma. Ann R Coll Surg Engl. 1971;49:329–49.
11. Robertson JH. Dental splints. Proc R Soc Med. 1964;57:184.
12. Kelsey Fry W, et al. The dental treatment of maxillofacial injuries. Oxford: Blackwell; 1942.
13. Tong DC. An evidence based and historical review of war surgery of the face and jaws. Thesis submitted to the University of Otago, 2013.
14. McGill Faculty of Dentistry. Celebrating 100 years of dentistry at McGill; 2003.
15. Kelsey Fry W. 1889–1963. https://livesonline.rcseng.ac.uk/biogs/E005380b.htm. Accessed 12 Jun 2022.

# Remembrance of Things Past. Plastic and Reconstructive Surgery. Vol 35, No 1, pp. 5–13

11

Shahid R. Aziz and Samina H. Aziz

**Abstract**

World War I, "The Great War," brought to reality suffering, violence, and destruction that were new to the human experience. Trench warfare during World War I provided surgeons with new challenges in facial trauma and laid the cornerstone for modern-day oral and maxillofacial surgery. While many surgeons and procedures came to fruition as a result of the facial trauma generated during this time, Varaztad Kazanjian was one of the true pioneers. His stabilization of facial trauma using dental principles, bone grating techniques, and aseptic protocols laid the foundation for modern-day maxillofacial reconstruction.

**Keywords**

Trench warfare · Gillies · Kazanjian: Sidcup · Anna Ladd · World War I

S. R. Aziz (✉)
Division of Oral and Maxillofacial Surgery, Department of Otolaryngology, Hackensack Meridian School of Medicine, Nutley, NJ, USA
e-mail: azizsr@sdm.rutgers.edu; Shahid.aziz@hmhn.org

S. H. Aziz
Class of 2028, Barnard College, Columbia University, New York, NY, USA
e-mail: sa4186@barnard.edu

"Remembrance of Things Past" was published in 1965 in *Plastic and Reconstructive Surgery*. It was a reprint of Dr. VH Kazanjian's lecture to the New York University Department of Plastic Surgery. In this paper, Dr. Kazanjian reflected on his time as a dental student and later dental surgeon at Harvard Dental School, as well as his time in France during World War I. World War I, "The Great War," brought to reality suffering, violence, and destruction that were new to the human experience. It is an unfortunate truth that war often provides fuel for medical advancement. Trench warfare during World War I provided surgeons with new challenges in facial trauma management and laid the cornerstone for modern-day oral and maxillofacial surgery [1]. Kazanjian noted that the period between the two world wars could be considered a time of the most rapid progress in the history of medicine.

The Great War lasted from July 28, 1914, to November 11, 1918. It was a consequence of the assassination the Austro-Hungarian heir, Archduke Franz Ferdinand, in Sarajevo by Gavrilo Princip, a Bosnian Serb Yugoslav nationalist. The resulting Austria–Serbia conflict escalated into two competing alliances: The Triple Entente (Allied)—consisting of France, Russia, and Britain—and the Triple Alliance of Germany, Austria-Hungary, and Italy (Central Powers). After the sinking of American merchant ships by German submarines, the U.S. declared war on Germany on April 6, 1917. The Treaty of



S. R. Aziz, M. D. Turner (eds.), *Classic Papers and Pioneers in Maxillofacial and Oral Surgery*,
https://doi.org/10.1007/978-3-031-63246-4_11

Versailles brought World War I to an end, signed on June 28, 1919, in Versailles, France.

As noted above, Trench warfare was a novel approach to warfare. It provided protection to the soldier from bodily injury due to gunfire; however, the soldier's face was often exposed. In 1915, steel helmets were introduced, protecting to at least some degree from brain trauma, but the face remained bare. Further, the Great War introduced a new age of high-velocity ballistic use and injury. What resulted was a never-before-seen volume and severity of facial trauma—soft and hard tissue. It is estimated that 15% of all injuries were facial. Often this injury rendered the soldier alive, but with massive tissue loss. Consequently, this forced the evolution and laid the foundations for modern-day facial reconstructive surgery. The reconstructive efforts could be broken into two basic efforts:

1. Frontline triage and stabilization: Typically, the soldier was stabilized, facial fractures reduced, and facial soft tissue injury treated for infection and hemorrhage. Soldiers were then transferred away from the front to more sophisticated centers. The best-documented frontline efforts were by the Harvard Surgical Unit's maxillofacial team lead by Dr. Varastad Kazanjian.
2. Tertiary care centers away from the front lines where hard and soft tissue reconstructive surgery occurred. The best known of these were two
   (a) Sidcup—lead by Sir Harold Gillies
   (b) Berlin unit—lead by Professor Jacques Joseph

Kazanjian noted that prior to the Great War, most facial injuries were basic fractures secondary to interpersonal violence with fists, or from falls. The advances of ballistics as well as the automobile created much more severe injury that was not seen until the Great War.

## Frontline Care: Origins of the Harvard Unit

Kazanjian noted that Sir William Osler proposed that leading American and Canadian universities should provide the Allied Forces with medical services near the fields of battle. Harvard, Johns Hopkins, Columbia, and McGill Universities arranged for medical "units" to be part of the Royal Army Medical Corps of the British Expeditionary Forces in France. On June 26, 1915, Harvard sent to England the first of 3 surgical units led by Dr. E.H. Nichols and composed of 32 surgeons, 3 dentists, and 75 nurses (the subsequent 2 units were led by Dr. David Cheever and Dr. Hugh Cabot, respectively).

When the First Harvard Unit was being formed, Dr. Nichols requested that Dr. Eugene Smith, Dean of the Harvard Dental School, select three dentists for inclusion. Smith, in turn, nominated Dr. Varaztad H. Kazanjian, who was at the time Instructor in Mechanical (Prosthetic) Dentistry and a 1905 graduate of the School, to be the Chief Dental Officer of the Dental Department of the Harvard Unit. Dr. Kazanjian readily accepted and chose as his assistants Ferdinand Brigham and Frank Cushman, both graduating seniors from Harvard Dental School.

Varaztad Kazanjian (1879–1974) was a remarkable individual. Born in what is now Eastern Turkey, of Armenian heritage, he immigrated at age 16 to the United States to avoid persecution by the Ottoman Empire. Settling in Massachusetts, he later attended Harvard Dental School, graduating in 1905, and further trained as a prosthodontist. He then served as a faculty member at the dental school, in charge of the prosthetic department. His interests at the time focused on Cleft palate, facial trauma, and postresection deformities of the face and jaws. Kazanjian writes that "in those days prosthetic appliances were used to replace defects of the Jaws" [2]. He notes that dentistry was ideally suited to treat facial fractures because of the dentists training in occlusion. Reestablishing occlusion created the foundation for stabilizing facial fractures and also created the support for future bone grafting. Following World War 1, Kazanjian then completed his medical degree at Boston University and returned to Harvard as a Professor of Oral Surgery and the first Professor of Plastic Surgery. He is considered to be one of the founders of modern plastic surgery, though he never forgot his roots in dentistry (Fig. 11.1).

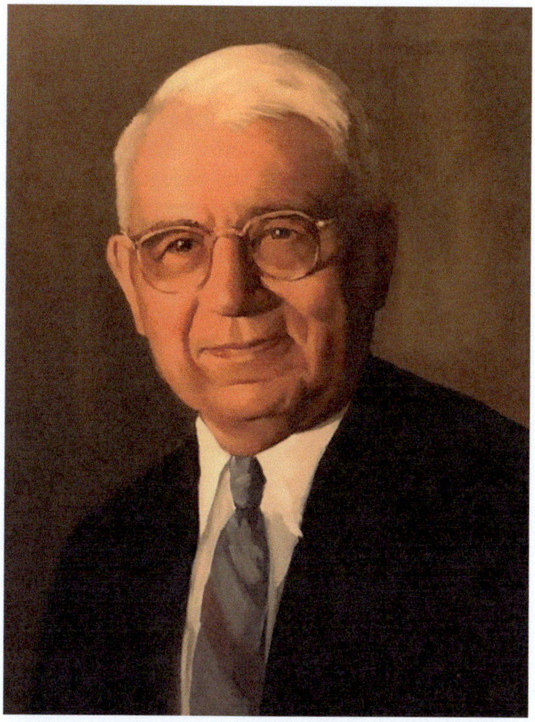

**Fig. 11.1** Portrait of Dr. Kazanjian in the lobby of Harvard School of Dental Medicine

The members of the Harvard Unit had a unique status in the Royal Army. Not British subjects, they were granted temporary honorary commissions in the Royal Army Medical Corps. The British War Office assigned this unit to Number 22 General Hospital at Dannes and Camier, France. Dannes and Camier were two hamlets located 14 miles south of Boulogne-sur-mer. No. 22 was 1 of the 5 base hospitals situated in Northern France. The hospital contained 1800 beds and was equipped with surgical and medical wards and operating facilities. The professional staff was housed in waterproof tents. These military base hospitals were adjacent to the front lines of fighting and sent "surgical teams" (teams of surgeons, anesthesiologists, and nurses) to the frontline casualty-clearing stations for emergent care, triage of the injured, and to facilitate a smooth transfer of the wounded to base hospitals.

Arriving in Dannes-Camiers, France, in July 1915, the Harvard dentists were the first to commence work. They were assigned one ward in the hospital and were kept busy with exodontia and prosthetic dentistry. Dr. Cushman later wrote in the Harvard Alumni Bulletin:

> Upon the arrival of the Unit in France, dental conditions were found to be much worse than expected. Until it became known throughout the district that fractures of the jaws were being treated by the Harvard Unit, much of the work was concerned with extraction of teeth and the making of artificial dentures. The most important phase of the work of the dental men in the Unit was, of course, the treatment of the cases of fractures of the jaws, and before the work was long underway, many cases of this sort were being brought in from the front and from other hospitals. The injuries were often very extensive, involving in addition to the jaws, other parts of the face and cranium. External wounds necessitate an entire change of procedure from the methods used in jaw fractures in civil hospitals. Owing to the drainage of Saliva through these wounds, the sepsis is widespread and persistent. Too much credit cannot be given to Dr Kazanjian for the masterly way in which these cases are being handled. Each new case requires the devising of special appliances to fit its particular needs; but this Harvard man is always found equal to every occasion [3].

One week after his arrival in France, Kazanjian created a plan for the Dental Department of the First Harvard Unit which consisted of two phases: (1) routine dental care for soldiers and (2) oral and maxillofacial surgery. When the 3-month term of the First Harvard Unit came to an end, the British War Office, cognizant of Kazanjian's excellent field work, requested that he stay on until the end of the war, or until he could train a successor. Kazanjian, while willing, was concerned about his absence from his position at the Dental School. Six surgeons of the unit petitioned Harvard President Lowell to allow Kazanjian to remain. Lowell cabled an affirmative response. Kazanjian then requested that the British War Office allow his assistants to remain and to provide better facilities in which to work. The British agreed and provided Kazanjian and his unit with better space and larger wards, relocating them to General Hospital 20.

Kazanjian wrote an article in the 1917 *British Medical Journal* detailing the daily activities of the Dental Department of the Harvard Surgical Unit. He noted that "soldiers who have received wounds of the face and jaws have for the first time been collected in centers for treatment." Advantages of this system included a nursing staff properly trained to efficiently handle maxillofacial injuries, the development of a dental laboratory that quickly produced splints and appliances necessary for treatment, and the opportunity to maintain a "comprehensive system of records from which deductions can be made on the complications, mortality, etc...." Cases were usually admitted to the dental department 2–3 days after injury. Kazanjian divided treatment into two distinct periods: the early period (usually 3–4 weeks after injury) and the convalescent period. The first, he considered essential for successful outcome. During this time, soldiers usually suffered from mental shock, toxic absorption from the wounds, exhaustion secondary to blood loss, and malnutrition secondary to inflammation of the oral cavity and damage to the masticatory apparatus. Further, it was during this period that patients were at highest risk for serious complications such as hemorrhage, bronchopneumonia, and generalized sepsis. The microorganisms involved in the septicemia were thought to be streptococcal; however, no positive identification was completed. Cellulitis was observed, originating from the wound, spreading over the face and scalp and accompanied by pyrexia. Bronchopneumonia was considered the most fatal complication. Some cases occurred suddenly, others gradually. Empyema and multiple abscesses in the lung were common. The pulmonary infections seemed to originate from the inhalation of septic material from the mouth. To prevent the onset of sepsis, initial treatment involved irrigation of the mouth at 2-h intervals during the day and night and swabbing of the soft tissues with iodine-soaked cotton. This was followed by surgical debridement of the wound under local anesthesia [4] (Fig. 11.2).

The second period was the convalescent period. During this time, definitive treatment of the oral and maxillofacial region was undertaken, including repair of the hard tissues by means of splints, construction of prosthetic appliances, and reconstructive operations for the repair of facial deformities. Based on his clinical experience, Kazanjian developed several basic principles for treating facial fractures: immediate immobilization of the fracture via the use of splints, reestablishment of the dental occlusion

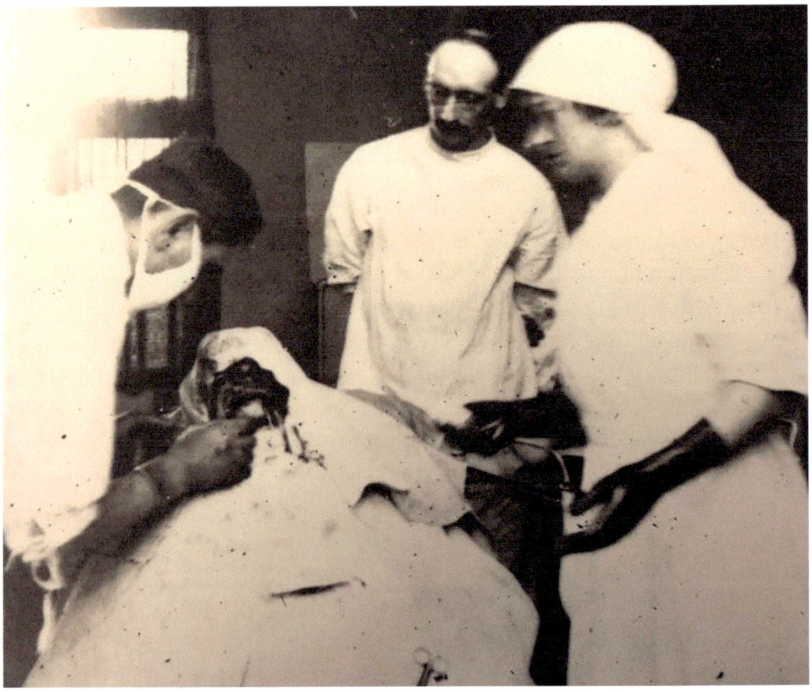

**Fig. 11.2** Kazanjian debriding a facial wound. (Courtesy Center for the History of Medicine, Francis Countway Library of Medicine, Harvard Medical School, Boston, MA)

as a guide for fracture reduction, early wound care and cleansing to minimize sepsis, and the control of blood loss. Kazanjian emphasized that early immobilization of fractures was the quickest and best means for recovery and, in turn, it reduced soft tissue inflammation, the risk of infection, and increased patient comfort. He noted that the primary function of splints was the fixation of bony fragments, which in turn provided support for overlying soft tissues. Nearly every splint was custom-made to suit each case. For cases of "ordinary" severity, standard splints were used to immobilize the jaw. In cases of extreme destruction of hard and soft tissues, Kazanjian found that intraoral splints were inadequate; an external support system composed of a series of vulcanite plates fitted over the forehead, and a headgear, was developed. This appliance stabilized the tissues of the mouth, nose, eyes, and neck. For extensive mandibular loss, Kazanjian created a sectional or folding artificial jaw; it acted as a framework for reconstructive operations and maintained the contour of the lower face. If the temporomandibular joint was involved in the injury, he placed a mechanical condyle to restore joint function. Before the Harvard Unit's arrival, one major flaw in the care of maxillofacial war injuries was the basic lack of dental training on the part of the military surgeon. Kazanjian noted: if a surgeon was called upon to treat a fracture of the mandible, in many instances he approximated the segments with wires or metal plates without regard to the occlusion of the teeth, while the dentist, in attending a similar injury, almost invariably applied intermaxillary ligation or immobilization of the jaw by some form of splint attached to the teeth which brought the jaws and teeth into natural occlusion. The key to Kazanjian's success was his training as a prosthodontist. He used dental occlusion as the guide for reduction of the fracture—a principle well known in the dental community but novel to the medical clinician. His work during the Great War with general surgeons brought to light this basic principle of fracture reduction in the medical community, bridging the "no-man's land" between medicine and dentistry [5].

With regard to management of the soft tissues, Kazanjian wrote that: "there does not appear to be much scope for primary suturing of gunshot wounds complicated by fracture of the jaw some advantages may follow accurate primary suture of those portions of the wound which involve the lip margins, the eyelids, the alar of the nose, portions of the external ears or the outlying tributaries of a radiating wound" [5]. He advocated the use of secondary suturing to lessen the amount of scarring. Immediate cleansing and debridement to minimize sepsis were most important for facial soft tissue trauma. Finally, in situations in which soft tissue reconstruction was required, Kazanjian used flap operations to cover deficiencies. He used primary and secondary suturing to reduce the region to be covered by the flaps and created an appliance to reproduce the bony tissue to serve as a framework to give a natural contour to the soft tissues of the face or neck and to prevent undue scar contraction.

During Kazanjian's 3.5 years in Dannes-Camiers, the Harvard Unit saw 3000 maxillofacial cases (Fig. 11.3).

News of the Unit's successful management of even the most complex facial injury spread throughout the Allied and German medical communities, and Kazanjian's methods soon became the standard of care for the soldier with oral and maxillofacial wounds. The British press dubbed Kazanjian the "Miracle Man of the Western Front" in honor of his surgical accomplishments. Kazanjian later wrote: "As I look back upon those busy years, it is apparent that the principles and methods evolved during World War for the treatment of maxillofacial injuries had far reaching influence on the surgical treatment of civilian injuries and of acquired and congenital deformities of the face and jaw as well as other parts of the body" [6]. The Harvard Unit was retired by the British Army on January 8, 1919. Kazanjian and Hugh Cabot were both invested by King George with the "Insignia of a Companion of the Order of St. Michael and St. George" at Buckingham Palace. (Fig. 11.4).

Upon returning from the Great War, Dr. Kazanjian rejoined the Harvard Dental faculty as professor of military oral surgery and, in 1919,

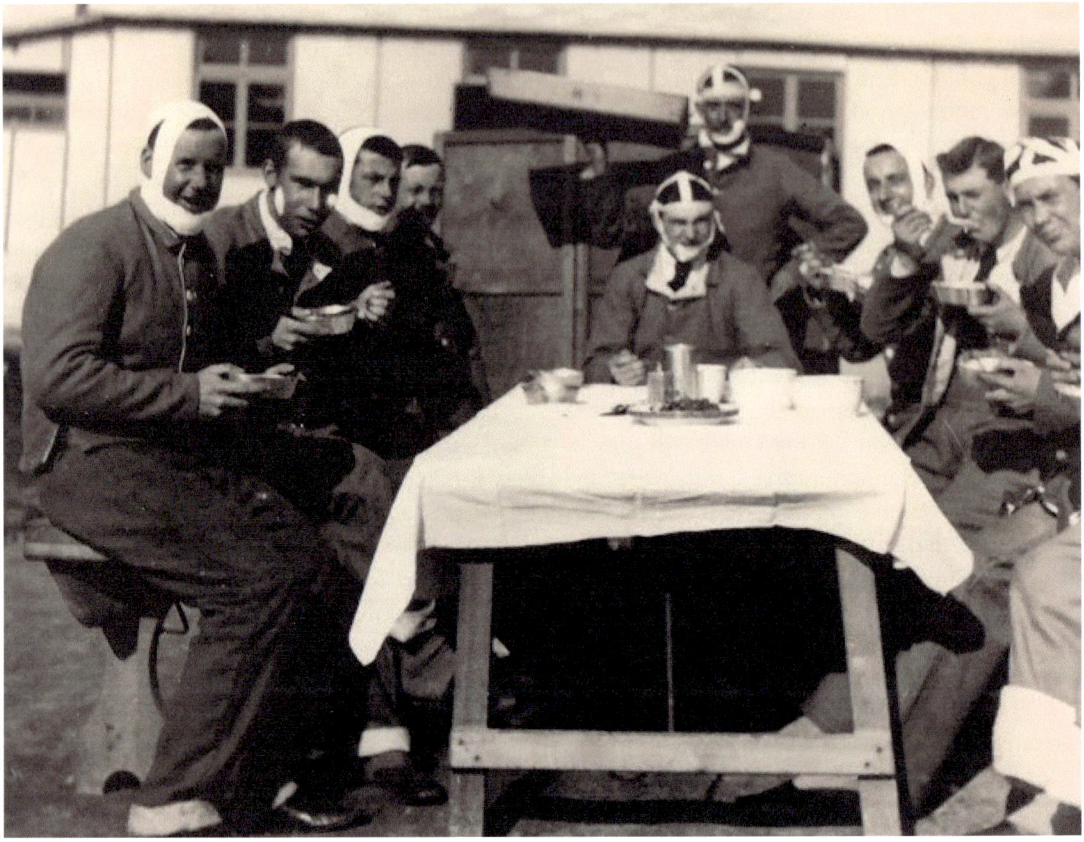

**Fig. 11.3** Patients of Kazanjian. (Courtesy Center for the History of Medicine, Francis Countway Library of Medicine, Harvard Medical School, Boston, MA)

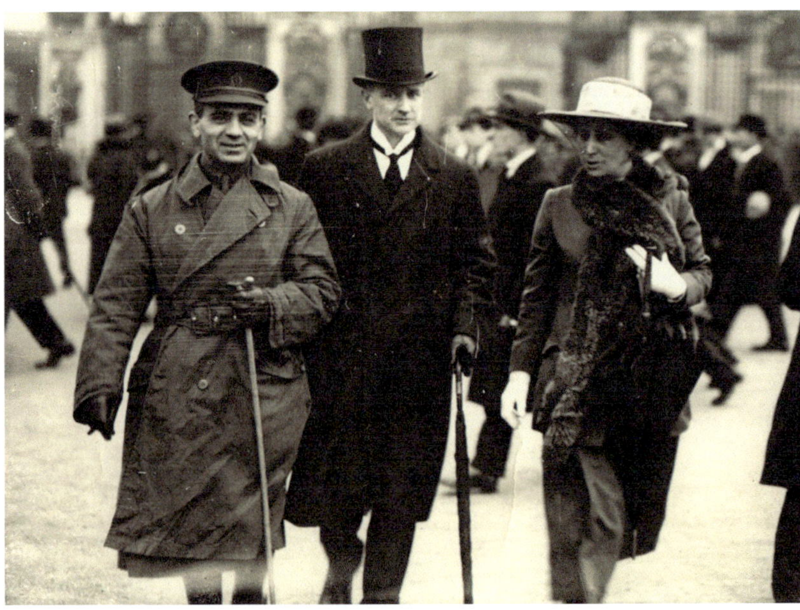

**Fig. 11.4** Kazanjian immediately after receiving his investiture outside Buckingham Palace. (Courtesy Center for the History of Medicine, Francis Countway Library of Medicine, Harvard Medical School, Boston, MA)

enrolled as a third-year student in Harvard Medical School. Kazanjian felt he should complete his medical training which would enable him to further his work and interest in facial surgery.

During medical school, Kazanjian was simply known as "the little dentist" who returned to finish medical school. None of his classmates knew of his significant accomplishments in the Great War. Toward the end of his fourth year, Kazanjian and his classmates attended a lecture by two British surgeons, who discussed their experiences with facial trauma. One of the surgeons recognized Kazanjian in the audience, and the two surgeons ran up and brought Kazanjian down to the front of the lecture hall, introducing him as the man who taught them exactly what they were lecturing on. From that point on, Kazanjian was considered a hero among his classmates.

After receiving his M.D. degree from Harvard, Dr. Kazanjian established a Boston-based practice of complex maxillofacial surgery, practicing until his 85th year. He maintained faculty positions at both Harvard Dental and Medical school, as a Professor of Oral Surgery and the first Professor of Plastic Surgery. Kazzanjian was a prolific author, writing 150 papers on maxillofacial surgery and co-authoring a pre-eminent text with his former student and colleague Dr. John Converse: Surgical Treatment of Facial Injuries in 1949. He championed multiple surgical techniques, perhaps best known for the vestibuloplasty technique he devised.

Kazanjian received honors and awards during his career, including: Special Honorary Citation of the American Society of Plastic and Reconstructive Surgery in 1951; an honorary Doctor of Science degree from Bowdoin College in 1952; the Honor Key Award of the American Academy of Ophthalmology and Otolaryngology in 1953; and the Chalmers H. Lyons Award of the American Society of Oral Surgeons in 1954. In 1962, the Kazanjian Visiting Professorship in Plastic Surgery at New York University Medical Center Institute of Reconstructive and Plastic Surgery was established. Dr. Kazanjian delivered the inaugural lecture entitled, "A Lifetime Experience in Plastic Surgery" which was later published as the paper highlighted in chapter.

Kazanjian was past president of the American Association of Plastic Surgeons, the American Society of Maxillofacial Surgery, and the New England Society of Plastic and Reconstructive Surgery. He was a fellow of the American College of Surgeons, the American Academy of Ophthalmology and Otolaryngology, and the American College of Dentists and a Diplomate of the American Board of Plastic Surgery. Kazanjian was an honorary fellow of the British Association of Plastic Surgeons in 1966 and an honorary fellow of the Royal College of Physicians and Surgeons in Glasgow, Scotland, in 1967.

In his tribute to Dr. Kazanjian, his former student Dr. Walter Guralnick quoted Dr. John Converse's reflection on Kazanjian:

> A man of great determination, though soft-spoken, with kindly eyes, one felt in his presence a vitality and keenness of perception. Imaginative and resourceful, he taught to improvise new methods rather than follow the conventional. 'Do it just right,' he would say, meaning in his laconic way (he preferred action to talk) that each patient's problem required an individual solution. Never did I hear him denigrate a colleague's work. His kindness, warmth, and modesty are legendary [7].

## References

1. Aziz SR. Harvard Dental School and the fight for the ideals of democracy. J Oral Maxillofac Surg. 2001;59:428–33.
2. Kazanjian VH. Remembrance of things past. Plast Reconstr Surg. 1965;35(1):5–13.
3. Cushman F. Work of Harvard Dental School graduates in France. Harvard Alumni Bull. 1916;28:614.
4. Kazanjian VH. The Department of Oral Surgery of the Harvard Surgical Unit. Br Med J. 1917;154:3.
5. Kazanjian VH. Observations on war surgery of the face and jaws. Dental Cosmos. 1920;62:283.
6. Converse JM. The extraordinary career of Dr Kazanjian. Plast Reconstr Surg. 1919;71:138.
7. Guralnick WC. Varaztad H. Kazanjian MD. N Engl J Med. 1975;292:806–7.

# 12 The Queen's Hospital, Sidcup. British Journal of Plastic Surgery, 6, pp. 247–249. 1953

Abrar Shamim and Shahid R. Aziz

**Abstract**

Wartime injuries to the maxillofacial complex during World War I provided the basis for advancements in both maxillofacial and plastic surgery. Dr. Henry Percy Pickerill joined the ranks of prominent New Zealand surgeons such as Harold Gillies through his work during the war, in addition to significant contributions to reconstructive plastic surgery, dental education, and various areas of research in both basic scientific and clinical contexts. Pickerill's short piece, "*The Queen's Hospital, Sidcup*" is discussed in the context of his contributions to the fields of plastic and maxillofacial surgery.

**Keywords**

Maxillofacial surgery · Plastic surgery · Henry Percy Pickerill · World War

A. Shamim
Department of Oral and Maxillofacial Surgery, Harvard School of Dental Medicine, Boston, MA, USA
e-mail: ashamim@mgh.harvard.edu

S. R. Aziz (✉)
Division of Oral and Maxillofacial Surgery, Department of Otolaryngology, Hackensack Meridian School of Medicine, Nutley, NJ, USA
e-mail: azizsr@sdm.rutgers.edu; Shahid.aziz@hmhn.org

Although New Zealand comprises only a fraction of the world's population, the specialty of facial plastic surgery was largely pioneered by its own, including Harold Gillies, Archibald McIndoe, Rainsford Mowlem, and the subject of this chapter, Henry Percy Pickerill [1]. Pickerill (Fig. 12.1)

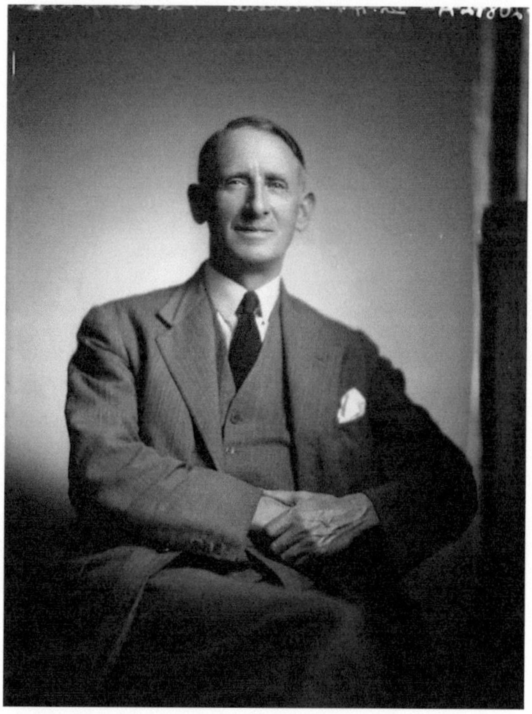

**Fig. 12.1** Henry Percy Pickerill (1879–1956) pictured on 23 March 1935. (Courtesy of the National Library of New Zealand [2])


S. R. Aziz, M. D. Turner (eds.), *Classic Papers and Pioneers in Maxillofacial and Oral Surgery*,
https://doi.org/10.1007/978-3-031-63246-4_12

became known as New Zealand's first maxillofacial surgeon and one of the Australasia's first plastic surgeons following his wartime service in the earlier part of the twentieth century. Much of his early work in plastic and maxillofacial surgery came about during the Great War, a time when developments in many surgical specialties, especially plastic and maxillofacial surgery, expanded rapidly due to the gruesome injuries seen during the war.

The UK training system for medicine and dentistry required independent routes of training, although some overlap was present at the University of Birmingham, where Pickerill decided to study in both fields. He completed LDS RCS (Licensee in Dental Surgery by the Royal College of Surgeons) in 1903 and BDS in 1904, both from the University of Birmingham. Then, in 1905, he completed MBChB (Bachelor of Medicine and Bachelor of Surgery), also referred to as MBBS, which is awarded in the UK and some other countries after 5 years of undergraduate–graduate studies and is the primary qualification in medicine. Later in life, also at the University of Birmingham, he completed an MD (in the UK, this is seen as an even higher qualification than MBBS/MBChB, which may be akin to a PhD track that is only available for qualified doctors to pursue), Masters in Surgery, and MDS (a higher degree in dentistry pursued by those pursuing research or academia) [3].

The Queen's Hospital in Sidcup is well-known historically as a center for treatment of injuries of the hard and soft tissues of the face, led by world-renowned Harold Gillies (one of the founding fathers of plastic surgery) and it was divided in such a way that surgeons would be in command of serving their respective countrymen; Gillies assigned the Canadians under Captain Fulton Risdon, the Australians under Colonel Henry Newland, and the New Zealanders under Pickerill [4]. As such, Pickerill's 1953 piece aptly titled "The Queen's Hospital, Sidcup" enlightens rich memory of his experiences at this massively influential hospital during the Great War. He described that the massive staff of the hospital had to labor wholeheartedly to keep their six operating rooms running, which were at maximum capacity daily; even so, Sidcup could still barely house healing patients. This hospital was the site of many developments, and Pickerill gives insight into why this may be:

> Although each section was self-contained and autonomous there was a common record office open to all; so that if the officer-in-charge of one section was too busy to go along and see how the officer-in-charge of another section dealt with some particular case, he could next day read all about it in the record office, and adopt the new method himself if he wished on the day following. Thus was progress speeded up [5].

Pickerill had the opportunity to independently develop his surgical skills and ideas for treating maxillofacial war injuries, which were abundant due to the nature of trench warfare; he was not specifically trained in the necessary surgical techniques. Over 200 servicemen were treated by Pickerill himself in the New Zealand section at Sidcup [6, 7], and it is likely that the large volume of cases and responsibility given to Pickerill to command the New Zealand unit allowed him to develop these new skills. He gained a reputation of having an excellent skillset and knowledge of plastic and maxillofacial surgery, which he would go on to bring back to Australasia after the war. For readers of the current day, learning surgical techniques without a knowledgeable mentor to learn from is an unfathomable (and unethical) way to increase exposure. However, Pickerill was required to develop in these techniques in the context of unprecedented war injuries at a time when maxillofacial and plastic surgery were still not developed and recognized fields and therefore did not yet have appropriate routes of training.

In his memoir of Queen's Hospital in Sidcup, Pickerill also described a common complaint from soldiers with facial injuries who previously underwent repair, who stated, "These blankety tin faces are no good to us. Can't you give us something that we can wash and shave and won't fall off in the street?" [5]. In his 1924 book titled *Facial Surgery*, Pickerill writes about the surgical repair of soft and hard tissue injuries, without the use of such tin replacement prosthetics, seen during the war (Fig. 12.2). Due to the rapid changes and developments to the respective fields during this time, it can be said that his book is one of the many additions to the literature which provided plastic and maxillofacial surgery with a literary foundation in the early twentieth century.

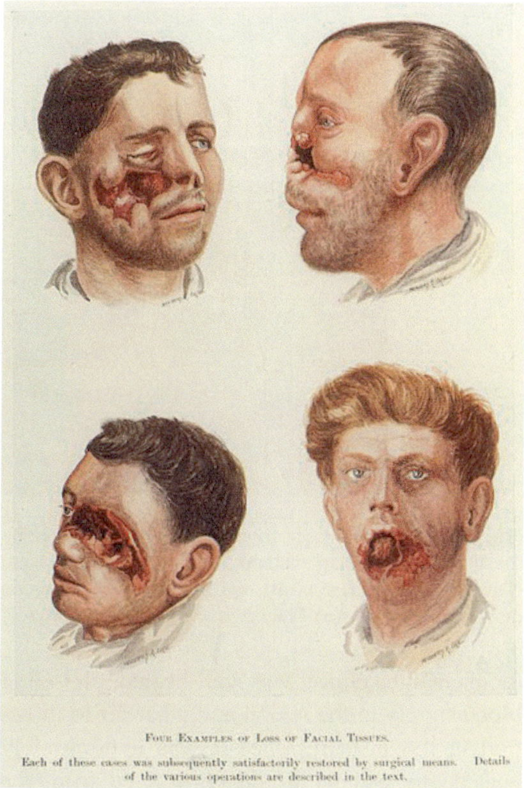


**Fig. 12.2** Title page illustrations in Pickerill's 1924 book *Facial Surgery* showing the faces of 4 men with loss of facial tissues from war injuries. Illustrations were done by Herbert R Cole. In this book, he describes the details of various operations, including autologous soft tissue grafting, to repair these types of injuries

Pickerill was part of a team that helped pioneer new techniques of tissue transfer [6]. There was a friendly rivalry between the surgeons at Sidcup; however, some authors write that this evolved into a competitive relationship between Gillies and Pickerill, in which each failed to acknowledge each other's role in wartime advancements [3, 6]. Pickerill did not mention Gillies' contributions in his 1924 book *Facial Surgery*. Nonetheless, one of the major advancements that came out of the Sidcup hospital was that of the tubed-pedicle flap, in which skin from neighboring regions to soft tissue injury of the face (such as the forehead or chest) was sutured into a tube-shaped cylinder and subsequently sutured into place of the soft tissue defect. It would remain anastomosed to the donor and

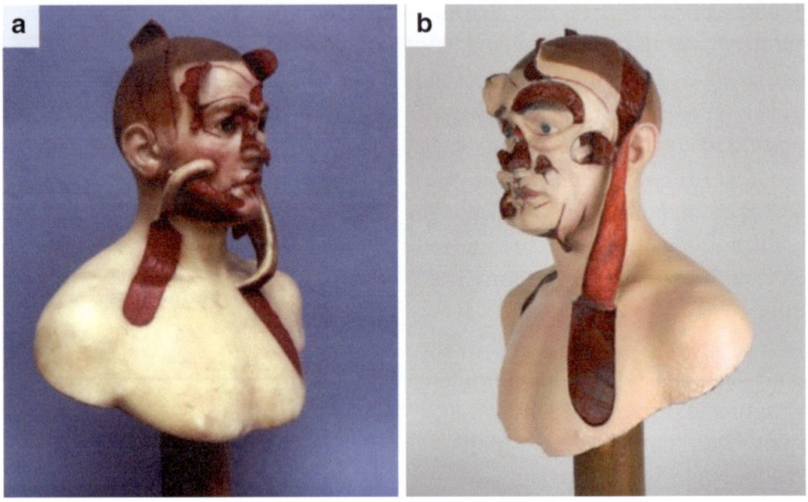

**Fig. 12.3** Pickerill's wax model created to demonstrate the tubed-pedicle flap method used to provide closure (therefore infection control) and blood supply to tissue defects of the face. (**a**) The original wax teaching model made by Sergeant Thomas H. Kelsey in 1917 [9] and (**b**) a 3D printed copy of the teaching model created in 2016, now held at the RCS Hunterian Museum. (Original figure courtesy of National Army Museum [7])

recipient sites until it was well-healed, providing blood supply to the region and a barrier to infection in the interim. Once it was appropriately healed, the pedicle would be severed from the donor site and the tissue expanded to substitute the soft tissue defect in the recipient site of the face. Gillies is often credited with this advancement, but it had also been independently published by Vladimir Filatov in Russia a few weeks prior [4]. Pickerill gained experience with this technique and others, and he employed them into his own practice; he also importantly advanced them in a pedagogical sense by creating wax models that were used for educational practices [8] (Fig. 12.2). The wax model shown in Fig. 12.3, along with others like it, returned with Pickerill to Dunedin, New Zealand, after the war [10]. Eventually, it found its way back to the UK and is now held at the Royal College of Surgeons Hunterian Museum Collection.

Pickerill is also credited with being one of the first to use bone grafts, from the ribs and elsewhere in the body, for the repair of hard tissue injuries of the face and jaws [3, 11]. Although it may be difficult to ascertain which developments were truly made by which surgeons, it cannot be debated that Pickerill brought many novel techniques in plastic and maxillofacial surgery from his wartime experience to Australasia.

## Life Before the War

Henry Percy Pickerill was born to Mary Ann Gurney and Thomas Pickerill in 1879 in Hereford, near the Welsh border of England; he was their only surviving son and grew up in this area [12]. He attended secondary school at Chandos School, Private Collegiate School of Hereford, and Hereford County College. In 1906, Pickerill married the former Mabel Louise Knott, with whom he had one daughter and three sons. As mentioned above, he received much of his post-secondary education at the University of Birmingham, including degrees in medicine and dentistry (LDSRCS, BDS, and MBBS/MBChB). He studied further to achieve higher degrees in these fields (MD and MDS). In 1923, he also obtained from the University of Birmingham a Master of Surgery, considered the highest master's degree in surgical science. His book *Facial Surgery* discussed previously was submitted to the University of Birmingham to attain this MS degree.

## From England to New Zealand, and Back

In 1907, Pickerill became founding Director and the first Dean of the Faculty of Dentistry in the University of Otago, Dunedin, New Zealand, when he was 28 years old. He had seen a flyer for this position while in England and decided to apply (Fig. 12.4). In 1917, he was assigned to return to the UK to serve in World War I as a captain in the New Zealand Medical Corps; he traveled back to the UK with the New Zealand Expeditionary Force on the troopship *Athenic* and established his own jaw department at the No. 2 New Zealand General Hospital at Walton-on-Thames, where he treated soldiers with facial injuries from the war fronts in Belgium and France [3]. He was then ordered to transfer his unit to The Queen's Hospital in Sidcup, where he led the New Zealand section.

After the war, he returned with his unit to New Zealand in 1919 and established the Facial and Jaw Department at Dunedin hospital until 1921 (Fig. 12.5). Fifty-nine of his patients returned to New Zealand with him on the *SS Tainui* and were to receive continued plastic surgery and rehabilitation following their war injuries. He also returned to his position of Dean of the University of Otago Faculty of Dentistry upon his return in 1919.

University of Otago,
Dunedin,
New Zealand.

SCHOOL OF DENTISTRY.

APPLICATIONS, with testimonials, for the position of Director of the School of Dentistry will be received by the Registrar of this University not later than 31st January, 1907.

Salary, £500 per annum.

Duties to begin 1st May, 1907.

Full particulars may be obtained from the undersigned.

W. A. MASON,
Registrar.

**Fig. 12.4** University of Otago call for applicants for Director of the School of Dentistry

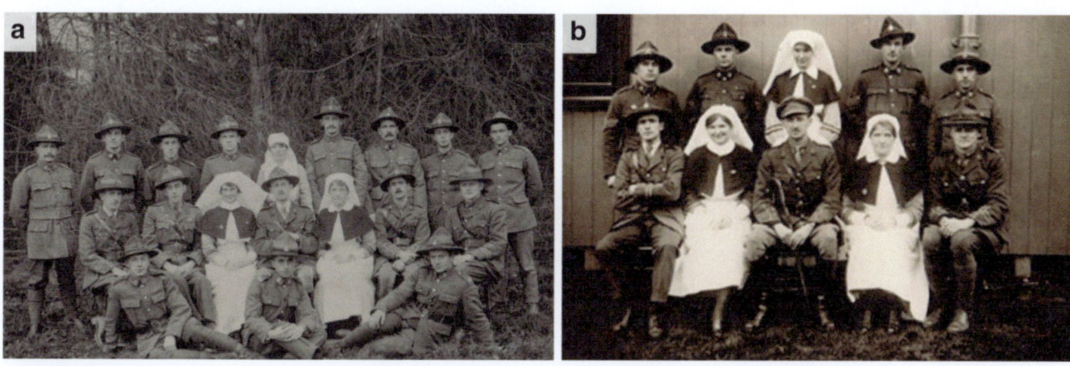

**Fig. 12.5** Lieutenant Colonel Pickerill pictured (center in both images) with his surgical, nursing, and technical teams (**a**), at the Queen's Hospital in Sidcup (1918) and (**b**), after the war at Dunedin Hospital, New Zealand (1919). (From the Pickerill Papers, Hockena Collections, Uare Taoka o Hockena, University of Otago, Dunedin)

## Academia

After finishing his medical and dental degrees in England, Pickerill was appointed a lecturer in dental pathology and histology at the University of Birmingham in 1906 [13]. As Dean at the University of Otago in New Zealand, Pickerill had many administrative responsibilities and a heavy workload [14], but he still managed to teach various subjects, including pathology, bacteriology, orthodontics, dental mechanics, and others. Pickerill conducted research in cariology, oral physiology, and oral/maxillofacial surgery [12].

By today's terminology, Pickerill embodied the title of "surgeon scientist" with many publications carrying his legacy in addition to his clinical work. He wrote extensively regarding his academic interests, which were many. Prior to the war, he was awarded the Cartwright Prize of the Royal College of Surgeons of England for his essay "The Prevention of Dental Caries and Oral Sepsis." He also published in 1912 a landmark book titled *Stomatology in General Practice: A Textbook of Diseases of the Teeth and Mouth for Students and Practitioners*. He published papers on many topics from dental enamel, salivary composition, immunity to dental caries, reconstruction of the face and jaws following trauma, and correction of congenital deformities such as orofacial clefts [13].

One of the Pickerill's great contributions to the field of dentistry will be remembered as his push for dental education to be borne out of university training, associated with medical education, rather than through a system of apprenticeship. He believed in a high standard of training, which he was able to achieve in New Zealand, and this has indeed become the reality of dental education in the twenty-first century which requires formal professional training with close integration with the biomedical sciences.

## Orofacial Cleft Hospital: Bassam

Pickerill established Bassam Hospital in Wellington, New Zealand, in 1939 to treat children and infants suffering from orofacial clefts (Fig. 12.6) and other congenital craniofacial deformities. Prior to establishing this hospital, he had given up his role at the University of Otago and was practicing plastic surgery in Australia. Pickerill utilized his experiences from the war to aid in infection prevention for the children, which included limiting visitors to the residences and not allowing visitors in the operating room. Uniquely, at this hospital all the nursing care for

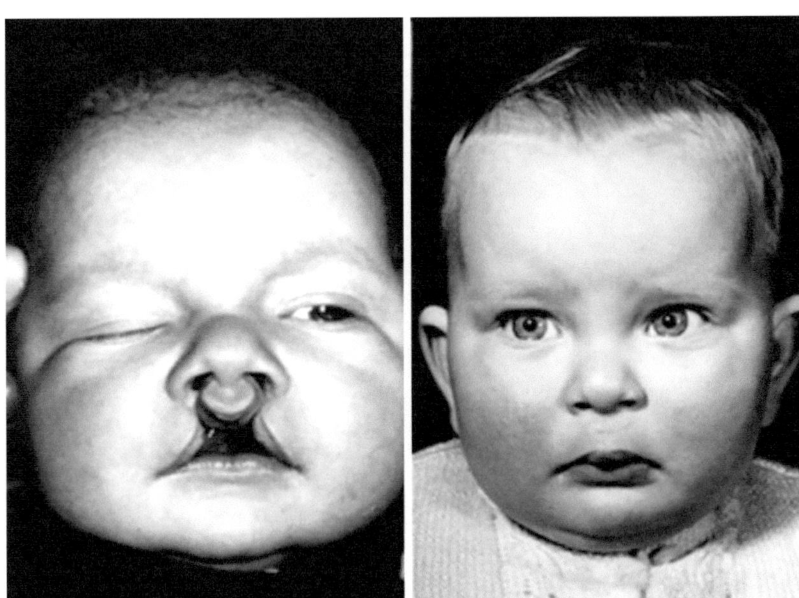

**Fig. 12.6** Pre- and post-operative photos of a child with bilateral complete cleft lip treated in 1947 by Pickerill and his second wife Cecily Clarkson. (From the Pickerill Papers, Hockena Collections, Uare Toako o Hockena, University of Otago, Dunedin New Zealand)

the children was done by their own mothers, except during surgery in the operating room. Additionally, it was the first hospital in New Zealand to give live-in accommodation for mothers to support mom–baby bond [13]. Pickerill contributed to and wrote about technical developments in cleft repair. At Bassam, he developed the triangular or zigzag graft to treat cleft lips [15]. He also published on this topic early in his career, in 1914 a book titled *The Anatomy and Physiology of Cleft Palate and New Method of Treatment* in which he proposed a two-staged method of cleft repair [16].

## Late Life

Pickerill was made OBE (Most Excellent Order of the British Empire) in 1919 and CBE (Highest Ranking Order of the British empire, excluding knighthood) in 1923. He resigned from University of Otago in 1927 and moved to Sydney, Australia, to practice plastic surgery at the Royal North Shore Hospital. Pickerill divorced his wife Mabel after moving to Sydney and met Cecily Clarkson, whom he would end up marrying a few years later [3] and had one child with. Although she trained under Pickerill and operated with him, Clarkson was not recognized by the medical profession because she held no postgraduate qualifications. It was with her that Pickerill established Bassam Hospital and also operated with at Middlemore Hospital near Auckland on the weekends, where they provided general plastic surgery, facial and jaw surgery, and cleft lip/palate repairs.

Pickerill died in 1956 in Pinehaven, New Zealand, and his ashes were taken to England and scattered near his birthplace in Hereford [13]. Many of his novel techniques and service to the nation of New Zealand were forgotten by the surgical establishment [3]; however, the authors of this chapter hope to keep his role in the histories of plastic and maxillofacial surgery, dentistry, and research alive.

## References


1. Zhang WY, Hallock GG. Gillies and Dunedin: the birthplace of modern plastic surgery. J Plast Reconstr Aesthet Surg. 2020;73:1012–7. https://doi.org/10.1016/j.bjps.2020.02.011.
2. National Library of New Zealand Henry Percy Pickerill. https://natlib.govt.nz/records/22911944. Accessed 7 Jul 2022.
3. Brown H. Henry Percy Pickerill—Pioneer Plastic Surgeon. https://www.kumc.edu/school-of-medicine/academics/departments/history-and-philosophy-of-medicine/archives/wwi/essays/dentistry/henry-pickerill.html. Accessed 27 Jun 2022.
4. Matthews DN. Gillies: mastermind of modern plastic surgery. Br J Plast Surg. 1979;32:68–77. https://doi.org/10.1016/0007-1226(79)90065-1.
5. Pickerill HP. The Queen's Hospital, Sidcup. Br J Plast Surg. 1953;6:247–9. https://doi.org/10.1016/S0007-1226(53)80036-6.
6. Pickerill and Gillies great war story. https://nzhistory.govt.nz/media/video/pickerill-and-gillies-great-war-story. Accessed 30 Jun 2022.
7. The birth of plastic surgery. https://www.nam.ac.uk/explore/birth-plastic-surgery. Accessed 7 Jul 2022.
8. Attwood B. "Remembrance Day 2019" by Adrian Reyes-Hughes. https://generic.wordpress.soton.ac.uk/medicallyspeaking/2019/11/08/remembrance-day-2019-by-adrian-reyes-hughes/. Accessed 2 Jul 2022.
9. RCS England RCSHM/Z 172—reconstructive surgical procedures, models (representations), busts. http://surgicat.rcseng.ac.uk/Details/collect/66094. Accessed 2 Jul 2022.
10. Alberti S. Treasures from the museums. Bulletin. 2014;96:36. https://doi.org/10.1308/rcsbull.2014.96.1.36.
11. Pickerill HP. Facial surgery. Edinburgh: E. & S. Livingstone; 1924.
12. Tong D, Bamji A, Brooking T, Love R. Plastic Kiwis—New Zealanders and the development of a specialty. https://jmvh.org/article/plastic-kiwis-new-zealanders-and-the-development-of-a-specialty-2/. Accessed 7 Jul 2022.
13. Brown H. Pickerill, Henry Percy. https://teara.govt.nz/en/biographies/3p25/pickerill-henry-percy. Accessed 7 Jul 2022.
14. Callister S. "Broken Gargoyles": the photographic representation of severely wounded New Zealand soldiers. Soc Hist Med. 2007;20:111–30. https://doi.org/10.1093/shm/hkl080.
15. Making Human Faces. Auckland Star 1927;LVIII:10.
16. Ilczuk-Rypuła D, Pietraszewska D, Kempa M, Zalewska-Ziob M, Wiczkowski A. Methods of cleft lip and palate treatment over the centuries—a historical view. Ann Acad Med Siles. 2017;71:399–406.

# Part III

# Twentieth Century Pioneers

# 13 Emergency Treatment of War Injuries of the Face and Jaws. Annals of Surgery. Volume 113, No 6. June 1941

Sara Mir and Neeraj Panchal

**Abstract**

Dr. Robert H. Ivy was a renowned oral and plastic surgeon known for his pioneering work in the emergency treatment of maxillofacial injuries as well as the development of a multidisciplinary team approach for treatment of children with cleft lip and palate. While serving as an officer in the Medical Corps during World War I, Ivy and his colleague published a highly influential article on the appropriate treatment of patients with war injuries of the head and neck, the basic principles of which still hold true today in the treatment of patients with maxillofacial trauma. Throughout his career, he continued to educate trainees at the School of Dentistry as well as the School of Medicine at the University of Pennsylvania. He received numerous awards and honors for his contributions to the fields of oral and plastic surgery including a certificate of appreciation from the War Department.

**Keywords**

Maxillofacial trauma · Reconstruction · Teaching · Pioneering · Robert Ivy

In the early years of World War I, a department was established in the 3rd London General Hospital by the name of "Masks for Facial Disfigurement Department" [1]. Some ruefully referred to it as "The Tin Noses Shop." This was where soldiers with severely disfiguring facial injuries went for fabrication of facial prostheses (Fig. 13.1) to cover areas of gross deformity. Trench warfare, which dominated World War I, made soldiers particularly susceptible to maxillofacial injuries [2]. This led to an urgent need for specialized medical centers as well as medical officers with expertise in treating injuries of the head and neck. Robert H. Ivy, an oral and plastic surgeon and officer of the Medical Corps, treated innumerable patients with traumatic maxillofacial injuries during World War I. In addition to becoming an expert in the treatment of such injuries, he played a major role in educating others about their treatment and strategies for improving outcomes. Many of the treatment principles that he outlined in his publications still hold true today in regard to treatment of patients with facial trauma [3, 4].

S. Mir
Oral and Maxillofacial Surgery Resident, University of Pennsylvania Health System, Philadelphia, PA, USA
e-mail: Sara.mir@pennmedicine.UPenn.edu

N. Panchal (✉)
Oral Maxillofacial Surgery, Penn Presbyterian Medical Center, Philadelphia Veterans Affairs Medical Surgery, University of Pennsylvania School of Dental Medicine, Philadelphia, PA, USA
e-mail: npanchal@upenn.edu



S. R. Aziz, M. D. Turner (eds.), *Classic Papers and Pioneers in Maxillofacial and Oral Surgery*,
https://doi.org/10.1007/978-3-031-63246-4_13

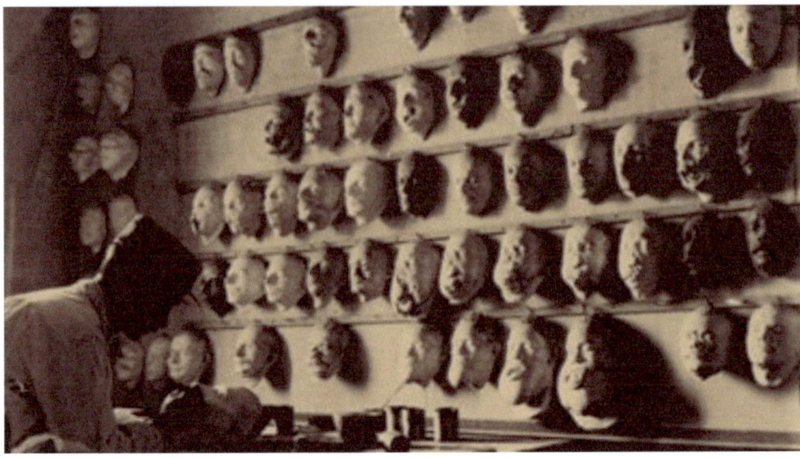

**Fig. 13.1** A studio for the fabrication of facial prostheses during WWI

In 1941, Ivy and his colleague Roy A. Stout, an officer of the Dental Corps, published a highly influential article on the appropriate emergency treatment of patients with maxillofacial injuries. The article, entitled "Emergency Treatment of War Injuries of the Face and Jaws," was read at the American Surgical Association meeting in West Virginia that same year. In the article, Ivy provides a stepwise guide on how best to approach maxillofacial injuries from initial stabilization to final reconstruction. He also underscores the importance of a systematic treatment approach and close cooperation between the medical and dental officers in order to optimize patient outcomes.

Ivy begins by describing appropriate first aid to wounded soldiers in the combat area, naming four conditions that require special attention as follows:

1. Arrest of hemorrhage.
2. Provision of adequate respiratory airway.
3. Temporary approximate reduction and fixation of bone fragments.
4. Provision of safe transportation from the combat zone to the hospital in the rear.

In cases of hemorrhage, Ivy explains that digital pressure may be applied over the vessel proximal to the wound to establish hemostasis. Additionally, he recommends that gauze packs be inserted into wounds of the maxilla or mandible and secured around the head with a "four-tailed bandage" (Fig. 13.2a) to maintain firm pressure. In cases of hemorrhage that cannot be controlled with pressure, he recommends a search for the bleeding vessel followed by ligation. Ivy goes on to explain the risk of airway compromise, especially in cases of bilateral unstable fractures of the maxilla and mandible. In these situations, he advises that an "emergency splint" should be placed to protrude the unstable segment of the maxilla or mandible (Fig. 13.2b), and if needed, anterior retraction of the tongue with a long suture or a large safety pin.

> Two tongue depressors are placed end-to-end and fastened by a third overlapping them in the middle with adhesive plaster. This piece is secured in a vertical position with a bandage passed around the head in the frontal region, with the lower end extending in front of the chin. A wire is passed around the lower front teeth or around the chin segment of the mandible and the end of the wire fastened to the lower end of the tongue depressor piece. The spring of this will effectively draw and keep the anterior segment of the mandible forward.

Ivy also emphasizes the importance of early treatment in the form of application of temporary fixation to maxillary and mandibular fractures for improved long-term outcomes. He describes a need for early, but conservative, debridement of wounds and reduction of fragments of the maxilla and/or mandible with bandages, elastic bands, or wires. He notes that "stabilization of the fragments helps to reduce pain and shock. It also assists in control of the tissues essential for the maintenance of a clear air passage, and reduces

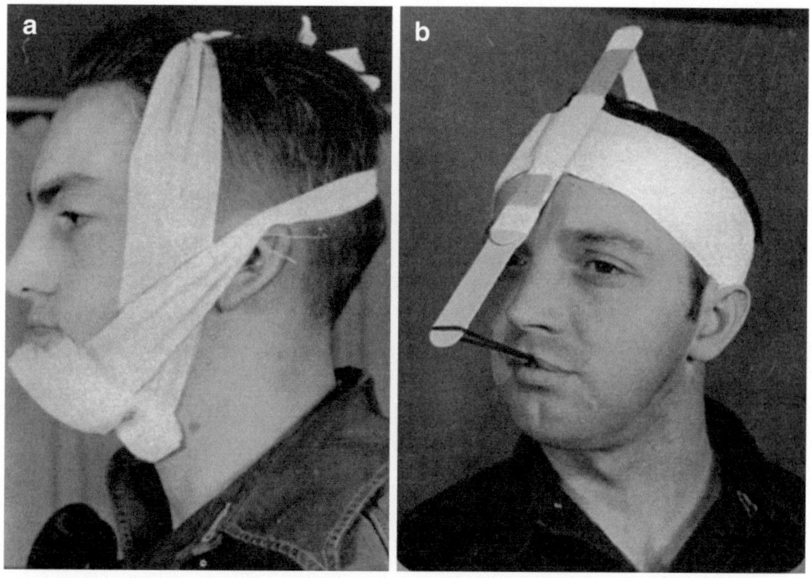


**Fig. 13.2** (**a**) (Right) The four-tailed bandage. (**b**) (Left) Emergency splint

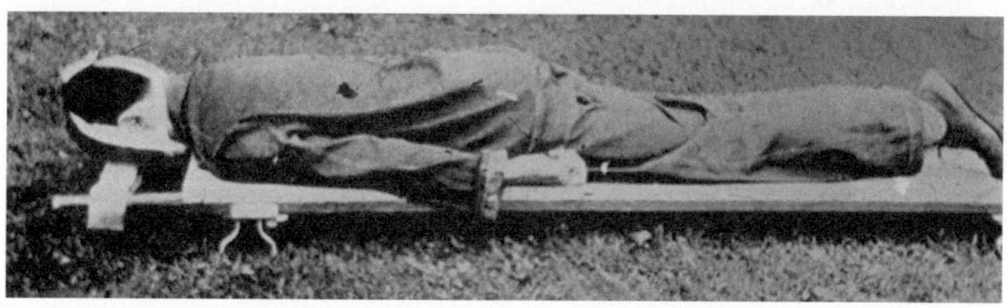

**Fig. 13.3** Transportation of the wounded soldier in the prone position

the danger of recurrent hemorrhage." He adds that any exposed bone within a wound should be covered with soft tissue whenever possible, but that this should be done after reduction and fixation of any underlying bone fragments. In cases of facial wounds that communicate with the mouth, he advises suturing skin to mucus membranes over exposed bone ends in order to reduce healing time.

Finally, Ivy goes on to discuss safe transportation of the wounded soldier from the combat zone to a hospital. He discourages inter-maxillary fixation prior to travel, likely out of concern for airway compromise. He goes on to recommend that patients with maxillofacial injuries who are unable to sit or stand should be transported in the prone position if there is any concern for airway obstruction (Fig. 13.3). He also underscores the importance of proper nutrition, analgesia, sedation, and prevention of shock in the (often long) transportation process to the hospital. He concludes by stating that the definitive treatment of patients with maxillofacial injuries depends heavily on the quality of preliminary care provided in the combat zone.

The oral and maxillofacial surgeon's current approach to the treatment of facial injuries has evolved significantly since the early 1900s. New technologies and an improved understanding of human physiology and microbiology have transformed the way in which we care for these patients. However, much of the principles outlined in Ivy's article regarding treatment of facial injuries still hold true to this day: the need for prompt evaluation of airway status and arrest of hemorrhage, the importance of early treatment for optimal outcomes, and the need for a team-based approach for complex injuries.

Robert H. Ivy was born on May 21, 1881, in Southport, England. His father, Robert S. Ivy, was a dentist, and his mother, Annie E. Cryer, was the sister of the renowned oral surgeon

Matthew H. Cryer [5, 6]. Ivy completed his early education at the Emmanuel School in London. At the age of 17, he emigrated to the United States and attended the University of Pennsylvania School of Dental Medicine. After completing his dental education in 1901, he served as the first dental intern at the Philadelphia General Hospital which, at the time, was the first hospital with a complete dental service, established by Dr. Matthew Cryer. Two years later, in 1903, Ivy enrolled in medical school at the University of Pennsylvania. During his third year of medical school, he briefly interrupted his studies to practice dentistry in China before returning to complete his degree in 1907.

Ivy cites his uncle, Dr. Cryer, as having a strong influence on his career choice since childhood: "I remember as a boy of 7 years (in 1888) being taken by my uncle, Dr. Cryer, to see my first surgical operation at the Garretson Clinic. It was for amputation of a crushed finger. I remember being a little frightened by the sight of blood and covering my face with my hands, but I peeked through my fingers." During his 3 years of dental school, Ivy lived at Dr. Cryer's house and assisted him with research on the anatomy of facial bones: "In a laboratory improvised on the third story of his house at Lansdowne, he [Dr. Cryer] cut hundreds of sections of human heads with a hand saw to gain access to the nasal accessory sinuses and other parts of the head, of which he made beautiful original photographs and lantern slides, right there in the attic room." In his publications, he refers to Dr. Cryer as his early mentor [7].

After completing his residency at the Episcopal Hospital of Philadelphia in 1910, Ivy opened an oral and plastic surgery practice in Philadelphia, the first of its kind. He also served as an assistant to Dr. Cryer who, at the time, was a professor of oral surgery at the University of Pennsylvania School of Dental Medicine. Ivy's interests, however, extended beyond the field of oral surgery and included urology and pathology.

When the United States entered World War I in 1917, Ivy was commissioned as Captain of the Army Medical Corps and served as an assistant to Vilray P. Blair, the commander of the U.S. Army corps of head and neck surgeons. Together, Blair and Ivy treated a vast number of patients with maxillofacial injuries. Notably, they also worked to train dentists and general surgeons in the treatment of injuries of the head and neck. Their goal, according to Ivy, was to "review the anatomy, the principles of plastic surgery, of splinting and the treatment of infections and sepsis of the face and jaw bones." Later on, Ivy was promoted as Major and served as the local consultant in maxillofacial surgery at the American base hospital in Vichy, France. Upon his return to the United States in 1919, he became assigned as the supervisor at Walter Reed General Hospital, one of the four major hospitals for the care of patients with head and neck injuries. In 1924, Ivy was elevated to Colonel in the Army Medical Corps. Throughout his career, he continued to work to educate practitioners about the treatment of facial injuries as well as pathology and infections of the head and neck [8]. For his work, he received a certificate of appreciation from the War Department and was buried with Military Honors.

Ivy's passion for teaching extended far beyond his time in the military. In 1920, he was appointed as a professor of maxillofacial surgery at the School of Dentistry as well as the School of Medicine at the University of Pennsylvania. He played an instrumental role in establishing the Department of Oral and Maxillofacial Surgery at Penn [9]. He also published countless articles and books, including a book entitled *Applied Anatomy and Oral Surgery for Dental Students*. In 1943, he went on to become professor of plastic surgery at the Graduate Hospital in Philadelphia and at the University of Pennsylvania. He served as a founding member of the American Board of Plastic Surgery, the American Association of Plastic Surgery, and the Journal of Plastic and Reconstructive surgery. Additionally, he went on to serve as an editor of *Plastic and Reconstructive Surgery*, an influential journal of the American Society of Plastic Surgeons.

Though the *Ivy loop*, an inter-maxillary fixation method commonly used by oral and maxillofacial surgeons today, is named after Ivy, he has disclaimed all credit for developing this tech-

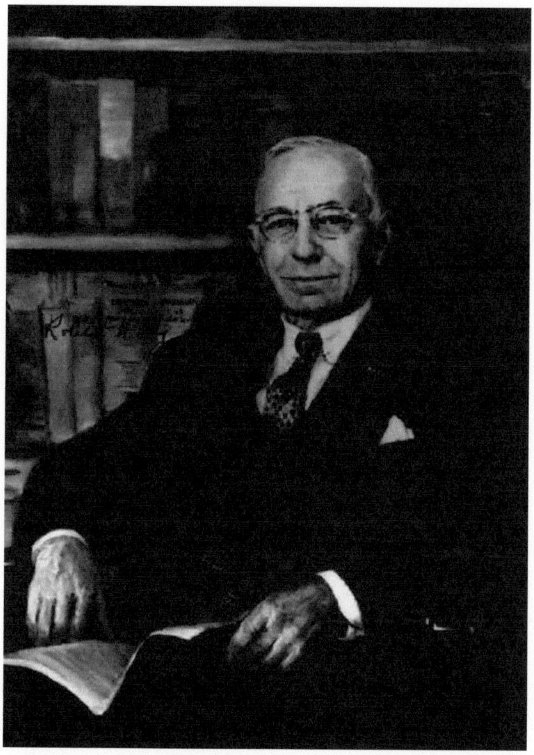

**Fig. 13.4** Dr. Robert H. Ivy

nique [10]. He has specified that all credit is due to his colleague, Colonel Robert T. Oliver of the US Army Dental Corps for developing the Ivy loop initially. Instead, he states his preference that the "real" Ivy loop should refer to the tubed pedicle flap used for reconstructing soft tissue defects of the cheek which Ivy developed and published in the *Journal of Plastic and Reconstructive Surgery* in 1949 [11].

After retiring from active practice, Ivy continued to work as a consultant to the Pennsylvania Department of Health for its cleft palate program. Perhaps his most notable accomplishment is the development of the multidisciplinary team approach for treatment of children with cleft lip and palate. Ivy received numerous awards and honors for his contributions to the fields of oral and plastic surgery throughout his career. The *Robert H. Ivy Pennsylvania Plastic Surgery Society* was formed in 1954. Dr. Ivy's portrait (Fig. 13.4) currently hangs in the Department of Plastic Surgery at the hospital of the University of Pennsylvania.

## References


1. Alexander C. Faces of war. Smithsonian Magazine. 2007. https://www.smithsonianmag.com/arts-culture/faces-of-war-145799854. Accessed 17 Dec 2021.
2. Strother EA. Maxillofacial surgery in World War I: the role of dentists and surgeons. J Oral Maxillofacial Surg. 2003;61:943–50. https://doi.org/10.1016/s0278-2391(03)00290-8.
3. Ivy RH, Stout RA. Emergency treatment of war injuries of the face and jaws. Ann Surg. 1941;113:1001–9.
4. Stelnicki EJ, Young VL, Francel T, Randall P, Vilray P. Blair, his surgical descendants, and their roles in plastic surgical development. Plast Reconstr Surg. 1999;103(7):1990–2009. https://doi.org/10.1097/00006534-199906000-00030.
5. Robert H. Ivy Pennsylvania Plastic Surgery Society: history of Ivy Society Part I. https://www.ivysociety.org/about.html. Accessed 20 Dec 2021.
6. Obituaries: Dr. Robert H. Ivy. The Pocono Record. 1974;12.
7. Ivy RH. Some early history in the development of oral surgery as a specialty. J Oral Surg. 1966;24:201–8.
8. Philadelphia (Pa.) Hospital of the Protestant Episcopal Church. Medical and surgical reports of the episcopal hospital, vol 1. Press of W.J. Dornan, Michigan;1913.
9. Oral and Maxillofacial Surgery Department History. https://www.pennmedicine.org/departments-and-centers/oral-and-maxillofacial-surgery/about-us/history. Accessed 15 Dec 2021.
10. Aziz SR. The person behind the name. J Oral Maxillofacial Surg. 1997;55:847–50.
11. Ivy RH. Single tubed pedicle in the form of a loop (letter to the editor). Plast Reconstr Surg. 1970;45:601.

# 14 Traumatic Mandibular Condylar Fracture Dislocations. Effect on Growth in the Macaca Rhesus Monkey. American Journal of Surgery, Volume 100. December 1960

Aram J. Keteyian and Paul A. Covello

**Abstract**

Born in 1924 in Waco, Texas, Dr. Robert V. Walker spent a lifetime deeply engaged in athletics and oral and maxillofacial surgery (OMS). His career helped define the role of the maxillofacial surgeon. Dr. Walker's career launched with the completion of a 2-year residency in OMS at Parkland Memorial Hospital, from which he graduated in 1956. Ultimately elected as the Chief of OMS at Parkland Memorial Hospital, he fostered the integration with the University of Texas Southwestern Medical School, laying the foundation to establish OMS as the primary service for the management of facial trauma. The landmark study presented in this chapter outlines the healing capabilities of the mandibular condyle and treatment protocols aimed at achieving optimal form and function. Dr. Walker's career has had a lasting influence on the field of OMS. Numerous surgeons have utilized the teachings of Dr. Walker to carve their own paths, and many maintain academic positions to this day. Briefly summarized in this chapter, Dr. Robert V. Walker's legacy will undoubtedly persist for generations to come.

A. J. Keteyian · P. A. Covello (✉)
Department of Oral and Maxillofacial Surgery, Geisinger Health System, Danville, PA, USA
e-mail: ajketeyian@geisinger.edu; pcovello@geisinger.edu

**Keywords**

Robert V. Walker · Oral and maxillofacial surgery · Mandibular condylar fracture · Mandible · Facial trauma · History

In the early stages of developing a consensus protocol for the treatment of mandibular condylar fractures, a distinct dynamic existed among providers with regard to potential therapies. One group held staunch beliefs about conservative management, whenever possible. The second group believed that surgical reduction was more appropriate for both pediatric and adult patients in most cases. The effect these fractures might have on the cartilaginous growth center for the younger patient population mandated a need to determine an optimized approach to management, as the literature was void of such information. In an effort to establish evidence-based treatment protocols, Dr. Robert V. Walker (Fig. 14.1) studied the healing of surgically reduced condylar fractures in young Macaca rhesus monkeys over a period of 16.5–20 months, post-operatively [2]. His efforts, outlined in his work, "Traumatic Mandibular Condyle Fracture


S. R. Aziz, M. D. Turner (eds.), *Classic Papers and Pioneers in Maxillofacial and Oral Surgery*,
https://doi.org/10.1007/978-3-031-63246-4_14

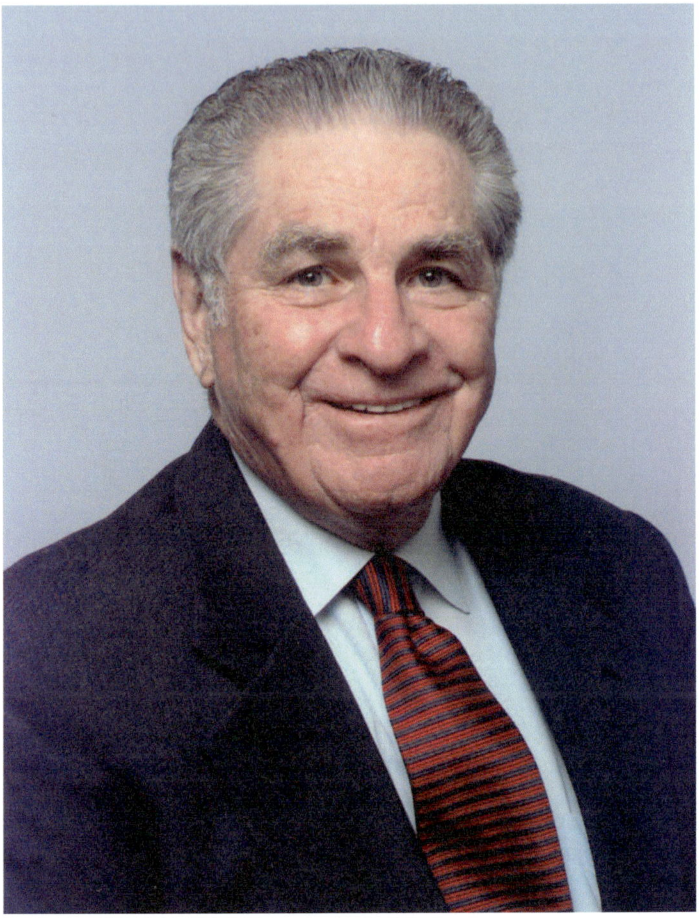

**Fig. 14.1** Dr. Robert V. Walker, Class of 1945, studied pre-dentistry at the Agricultural and Mechanical College of Texas. In 2004, he was honored with induction into the Texas A&M College of Science Academy of Distinguished Former Students [1]

Dislocations," elucidated several key concepts regarding post-operative wound healing, which provided an understanding of the healing capabilities of the mandibular condyle.

Conventional management of dislocated condylar fractures typically involved some level of stabilization (i.e., intermaxillary fixation) over an arbitrary amount of time. A new area of exploration revolved around the theoretical probability that the animal could form a functional articulation of a newly formed neo-condyle, regardless of the type of treatment or the length of stabilization. Of nine total subjects, only the control underwent closed reduction and complete immobilization of the mandible post-operatively; the remaining subjects were not immobilized. Each procedure was carried out in similar fashion, utilizing the previously well-described Risdon approach with careful re-attachment of the masseter muscle followed by layered closure [2, 3]. Once the appropriate amount of time had passed post-operatively, microscopic specimens of the condyle were obtained at varying intervals in order to qualitatively analyze the epiphyseal cartilage.

In this study, Dr. Walker remarked that, "a completely distinct fibrous covering, zone of cartilage, zone of ossification, and bone existed in the usual condylar, microscopic, anatomic order" [2]. This observation, along with the radiographic data obtained, provided strong evidence of the proclivity of the cells at the mandibular growth centers to regenerate with anatomically similar and functional neo-condyles. The results were noted regardless of the type of treatment rendered or the position of the fractured condyle, post-operatively. An evident drawback to immediate mobilization was the medial angulation of the mandibular angle, likely a result of "taxing the proper healing of reattachment" of the masseter due to the lack of post-operative fixation. Notably, however, each animal was still able to maintain a stable occlusion without a visible shift or open-bite.

An in-depth study of the microscopic activity of the mandibular condylar head sections demonstrated convincing evidence of the regenerative potential of the epiphyseal cartilage. As a result, both conservative and surgical management of these injuries were considered reasonable and justifiable. Furthermore, this study marked the beginning of a paradigm shift trending toward early mobilization or immediate functional rehabilitation of the mandible. Dr. Walker's important conclusions stating, "conservative management of such fractures in these young animals can yield results equally as satisfying as these attained through direct reduction and fixing of the condyle in anatomic alignment," reinforced the well-known healing potential of young patients and their remarkable ability to overcome devastating injuries with excellent functional results, in most cases [2].

A landmark work in the field, Dr. Walker's efforts to elucidate a physiologic basis that would solidify treatment protocols for displaced condylar fractures led the way for countless new studies and theories, all aimed at optimizing functional and anatomic outcomes in patients with mandibular condylar fractures.

## Early Life, Academics, and the Military

Born on September 21, 1924, in Waco, Texas, Dr. Robert V. Walker was one of the two children of father William Dedrick Walker and Ann Harrold Peevey [4]. His father, a farmer, and mother, a teacher, Dr. Walker was raised on a farm in Satin, Texas. He was fortunate to enjoy all the benefits of an outdoor lifestyle, including the time spent honing his athletic skills, particularly as they related to his love for baseball. The endless hours of rigorous practice and discipline, in addition to his academic prowess, led Dr. Walker to Texas A&M in 1941, where he studied a pre-dental curriculum and earned a place on the baseball team. Remarkably, he obtained both freshman and varsity letters while also being awarded the prestigious award of "Best-Drilled Cadet" for his admirable discipline and determination [4, 5].

Arriving to Texas A&M just prior to the beginning of World War II inevitably led to a disruption in the continuity of his collegiate years. In 1943, he entered the U.S. Army Field Artillery and in 1944 was serendipitously assigned to the Baylor College of Dentistry. During his time in dental school, he continued to pursuit his love for baseball. He played professionally for the local team in Dallas, TX, which culminated into signing a contact with the Chicago Cubs in 1946. After Spring training with the Tulsa Oilers, a Cubs affiliate, he ultimately decided to return to Waco, TX, to complete his dental training. In 1947, once the war ended and he was discharged from the U.S. Army, he married his wife Emily and earned his DDS degree [4].

Upon the completion of his dental education, Dr. Walker opened a local practice in Waco, TX, where he resided and practiced for 4 years. In 1951, he was called to return to service in the U.S. Army during the emergence of the Korean War. Fortunately, and in part because of his tremendous talent for baseball, he was assigned to the Brooke Army Medical Center in San Antonio, TX—one of the only three Army medical centers designated specifically as a Maxillofacial Injury Care Center. At Brooke Army Medical Center, as a general dentist and athlete, he gained a significant exposure to a great volume and wide variety of maxillofacial trauma. Over 28 months, he grew enamored with the specialty and eagerly turned his academic and professional efforts toward becoming an oral and maxillofacial surgeon [1].

Upon his discharge from the U.S. Army in 1953, Dr. Walker enrolled at the University of Pennsylvania Graduate School of Medicine in Philadelphia, where he studied for 2 years. While there, he maintained his fervor for maxillofacial surgery. Following graduation, he relocated to Dallas, TX, where he completed a two-year residency in oral and maxillofacial surgery at Parkland Memorial Hospital (PMH, Fig. 14.2), graduating in 1956 [1]. A truly defining period for him, the experience forged his personal goals while simultaneously affording him opportunities to practice and perfect his craft as an oral and maxillofacial surgeon in a busy academic center. Subsequently, he was offered a full-time faculty position at the University of Texas Southwestern Medical School. Within the Department of Surgery, he created the Division of Oral and Maxillofacial Surgery, for which he served as Professor and Chairman until 1984. Even after his retirement in 1997, he maintained an active role in the department, admirably spending his time and effort teaching students, interns, residents, and faculty of the program. Given the prestige and reputation he built for the program, a network of "Parkland Alums" would eventually develop, connecting former residents all over the country, leading back to the ties they shared with the esteemed Dr. Walker. Perhaps as impressive as his other accomplishments, he also maintained the status of Professor Emeritus throughout the entirety of his retirement.

In addition to the substantial impact Dr. Walker had on the specialty locally, regionally, and nationally, his efforts to teach and expand his beloved profession notably extended internationally, particularly in South America. In 1962, he held the honor as a founding member of the International Association of Oral and Maxillofacial Surgeons, an organization for which he would ultimately serve as President [4]. As a distinguished pioneer in the field of oral and maxillofacial surgery, he was later granted Honorary Fellowships from the Royal College of Surgeons of Ireland in 1973 and the Royal College of England in 1984 [1]. The devout efforts he made to developing and advancing the specialty of oral and maxillofacial surgery in South America fostered an international exchange of knowledge, students, and mentors. Consequently, students, residents, and faculty would disseminate to their home countries, where they would pass on and expand the teachings of Dr. Walker [4]. Always in the forefront of his mind was the sense of belonging to an institution. Specifically, he believed through willing and meaningful participation, the impact and joy of the profession would be spread in the most lasting and applicable manner. His devotion to involvement in professional organizations remained throughout the entirety of Dr. Walker's profound and remarkable career as an oral and maxillofacial surgeon.

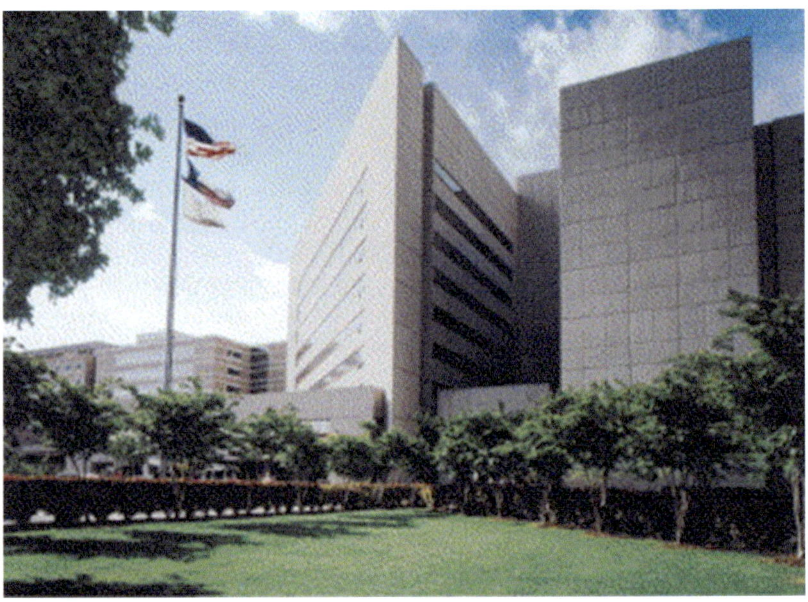

**Fig. 14.2** Parkland Hospital [6]

## Leadership

Refined through a lifetime of unique challenges and experiences, including athletics, wartime military training, education in dentistry and medicine, and a career in hospital-based academic surgery, Dr. Walker possessed an inherent mastery and passion for leadership. He truly understood the importance of advocating for oral and maxillofacial surgery, developing groups of individuals who would long continue his mission. As such, he served in several leadership roles, including President for the following organizations: the Southwest Society of Oral Surgeons (1973), the International Association of Oral and Maxillofacial Surgeons (1989–1992), the American Association of Oral and Maxillofacial Surgeons (AAOMS, 1974), the American Board of Oral and Maxillofacial Surgery (ABOMS, 1969), and the American Trauma Society [4]. As an example of his vision and innovation, Dr. Walker and three of his three colleagues lead the effort to obtain authorization from the American Dental Association to update the organization's name to Oral and Maxillofacial Surgery. Due to his contributions to the specialty, the AAOMS annual meeting was dedicated to him in 1987 [5].

As mentioned previously, Dr. Walker's impact on the specialty resounded internationally, garnering distinct recognition and praise. Working with British colleagues, he helped organize the first international conference in oral surgery, held at the Royal College of Surgeons in London in 1962. The success of the conference eventually led to the founding of the International Association of Oral and Maxillofacial Surgeons, established in Copenhagen, Denmark in 1965. He has also been recognized and appreciated for his work with colleagues in South America, the Philippines, and Japan throughout his career [4]. As a testament to his wisdom, experience, and stellar reputation in the field of oral and maxillofacial surgery, he served the Supreme Court of Arkansas as an expert witness in a case of malpractice in Little Rock [6]. A more expansive list of the items of recognition that Dr. Walker received is detailed in Table 14.1.

Dr. Walker was inducted into the Hall of Fame at the Baylor College of Dentistry—now known as Texas A&M Health Science Center—in 1999

**Table 14.1** Dr. Walker's notable items of recognition, listed in reverse chronological order [1]

| |
|---|
| • Texas Dental Association Gold Medal for Distinguished Service, 2003 |
| • Dallas County Dental Society Lifetime Achievement Award, 2002 |
| • Induction into the Baylor College of Dentistry Hall of Fame, 1999 |
| • William S. Stone Award for Contributions to Injury Prevention and Control, American Trauma Society, 1998 |
| • Establishment of the Robert V. Walker Society (for Planned Giving), Oral and Maxillofacial Surgery Foundation, 1997 |
| • Honorary Fellowship, International Association of Oral and Maxillofacial Surgery, Kyoto, 1997 |
| • Establishment of the Robert V. Walker Chair in Oral and Maxillofacial Surgery, the University of Texas Southwestern Medical Center, Dallas, 1992 |
| • Distinguished Service Award, American Trauma Society, 1992 |
| • Donald B. Osbon Award for Outstanding Educator, American Association of Oral and Maxillofacial Surgeons, Section on Education, 1990 |
| • Alpha Omega Alpha, Honorary Medical Society, 1988 |
| • W. Harry Archer Distinguished Achievement Award, American College of Oral and Maxillofacial Surgeons, 1988 |
| • Dedication of the American Association of Oral and Maxillofacial Surgeons Annual Meeting to Robert V. Walker, 1987 |
| • Distinguished Alumnus Award, Baylor College of Dentistry, 1985 |
| • Elected as Fellow in Dental Surgery Royal College of Surgeons of England, 1984 |
| • Distinguished Service Award, American Association of Oral and Maxillofacial Surgeons, 1981 |
| • Elected as Fellow of Faculty of Dentistry Royal College of Surgeons of Ireland, 1973 |
| • Omicron Kappa Upsilon, 1947 |

[1]. He was a founding member and past president of the Texas A&M Medical-Dentistry Society, a member of the Texas Aggie Corps of Cadets Association, the Texas A&M Foundation, and the 12th Man Foundation. He and his wife have been honored by the Emily and Robert Walker Endowed Scholarship in Science, which was eventually followed by the Emily and Robert Walker Endowed Lectureship in Biology in 1995 [1]. In 2004, he was inducted into the Texas A&M College of Science Academy of Distinguished Former Students. Through his efforts as a Professor of Surgery in the Division of Oral and Maxillofacial Surgery at the University of Texas Southwestern Medical Center, Dr. Walker successfully developed what has been considered a top-tier training program, which has withstood the test of time. The residency program he created remains in high regard among rising and active oral and maxillofacial surgeons.

## An Enduring Legacy

Ultimately, the legacy of Dr. Robert V. Walker extends through and beyond his contributions to oral and maxillofacial surgery. Elected as the Chief of Oral and Maxillofacial Surgery at Parkland Memorial Hospital in 1958, he saw the opening of the University of Texas Southwestern Medical School, fostered its integration with Parkland Memorial Hospital—an association including the affiliation with John Peter Smith (JPS) hospital—and facilitated the rapid expansion of the department as the hospital elevated its status as a Trauma Center. He then laid the foundation to establish the Division of Oral and Maxillofacial Surgery as the primary service for facial trauma [7]. Subsequently, in 1967, he became one of the first surgeons to perform a Le Fort III osteotomy in the United States. Strategically, he recruited talented and prolific surgeons to the faculty, including Dr. Jim Bertz, Dr. Bruce Epker, Dr. Larry M. Wolford, and Dr. William H. Bell. Encouraged and supported by him, each flourished and contributed substantially to the advancement of the field of oral and maxillofacial surgery [7]. Most impressively, many graduates of the oral and maxillofacial residency program during the era of Dr. Robert V. Walker continued to academic positions, introduced Cleft and Craniofacial Surgical Care, and contributed to the advancement of the specialty at various programs across the country.

Dr. Robert V. Walker died on April 28, 2011, following a battle with pancreatic cancer. His vision, organization, and passion created a baseline of excellence in training, patient care, and surgical innovation in oral and maxillofacial surgery, which will serve as a metric that will persist as the field advances beyond what he imagined.

## References


1. Tribute wall, distinguished alumni: Dr. Robert V. Walker '45. The Association of Former Students. Texas A&M University Web site. https://www.aggienetwork.com/tribute/index/206-11/. Updated 2012. Accessed 11 Sept 2022.
2. Walker RV. Traumatic mandibular condylar fracture dislocations: effect on growth in the Macaca rhesus monkey. Am J Surg. 1960;100(6):850–63. https://doi.org/10.1016/0002-9610(60)90516-X.
3. Risdon F. Ankylosis of the temporomandibular joint. J Am Dent Assoc. 1933;21(11):1933–7.
4. The Dallas Morning News. Bob Walker Obituary. 2011. https://obits.dallasnews.com/us/obituaries/dallasmorningnews/name/bob-walker-obituary?id=10671130. Accessed 13 Sept 2022.
5. Wolford LM. The history of oral and maxillofacial surgery at Baylor University Medical Center. Proc (Baylor Univ Med Cent). 2004;17(1):35–41. https://doi.org/10.1080/08998280.2004.11927955.
6. Walker RV, Sinn DP, Ellis E. Oral and maxillofacial surgery, University of Texas Southwestern Medical Center/Parkland Memorial Hospital. J Oral Maxillofac Surg. 2006;64(4):571–5. https://doi.org/10.1016/j.joms.2006.01.004.
7. Ricalde P, Turvey TA. History of craniofacial surgery in the United States: the role of the oral and maxillofacial surgeon. J Oral Maxillofac Surg. 2014;76(9):1842–6. https://doi.org/10.1016/j.joms.2018.06.178.

# New Methods for Immobilization of the Mandible. Oral Surgery, Oral Medicine, Oral Pathology, Oral Radiology, and Endodontology. No 1, pg 98–106. 1948

**15**

Joel Friedman, Lindsay D'Amato, and Sophia Jelke

**Abstract**

Dr. Kurt Thoma was a quintessential academic surgeon—prolific clinician, author, and researcher. Thoma was a full scope oral and maxillofacial surgeon—with expertise in trauma management as well as oral pathology. Thoma was born in Switzerland and educated in Switzerland and the United States. He spent his career at Harvard, where he maintained a busy practice, authored multiple texts, and was a Professor of Oral Surgery at the University of Pennsylvania, Harvard, and Boston University.

**Keywords**

Mandible fracture · Maxillomandibular fixation · Facial trauma

The evolution of techniques for mandible immobilization that support fracture reduction and healing has progressed from the use of bandage wraps like the Barton bandage to current techniques that include many different options for internal and external maxillomandibular fixation. Mandible immobilization is a core component of facial fracture management in oral and maxillofacial surgery. Proper immobilization of the mandible allows for minimal forces on jaw fracture segments and helps minimize risk of nonunion in bone healing. It also helps to restore proper occlusion and function for the patient. One of the pioneering surgeons in the evolution of mandibular immobilization for the treatment of mandible fractures was Dr. Kurt Thoma.

In 1948, Thoma published the paper "New Methods for Immobilization of the Mandible" introducing different techniques for mandible immobilization in patients with inadequate dentition or edentulism: one method of external craniomandibular fixation and two methods of internal maxillomandibular fixation. Dr. Kurt Thoma contributed to the evolution of mandible immobilization by introducing different techniques for immobilization, especially in an edentulous patient or a patient with inadequate dentition, that enhanced stability of fracture reduction against forces from speech and mastication.

"New Methods for the Immobilization of the Mandible" by Dr. Kurt Thoma originally appeared in the journal *Oral Surgery, Oral Medicine, Oral Pathology, and Oral Radiology* in 1948. In the article, Dr. Thoma discusses external craniomandibular fixation and internal maxillo-

J. Friedman (✉) (Deceased) · L. D'Amato · S. Jelke
Department of Oral and Maxillofacial Surgery, Columbia University College of Dental Medicine, Columbia University New York-Presbyterian Hospital, New York, NY, USA
e-mail: ld2936@cumc.columbia.edu; sgj2118@cumc.columbia.edu



S. R. Aziz, M. D. Turner (eds.), *Classic Papers and Pioneers in Maxillofacial and Oral Surgery*,
https://doi.org/10.1007/978-3-031-63246-4_15

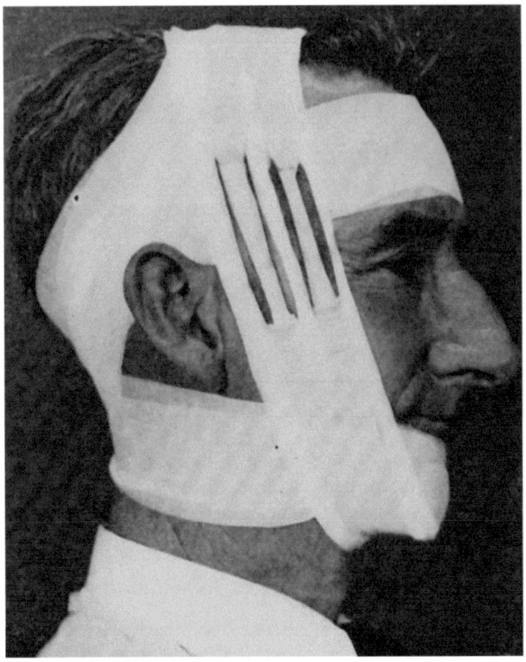

**Fig. 15.1** Barton bandage

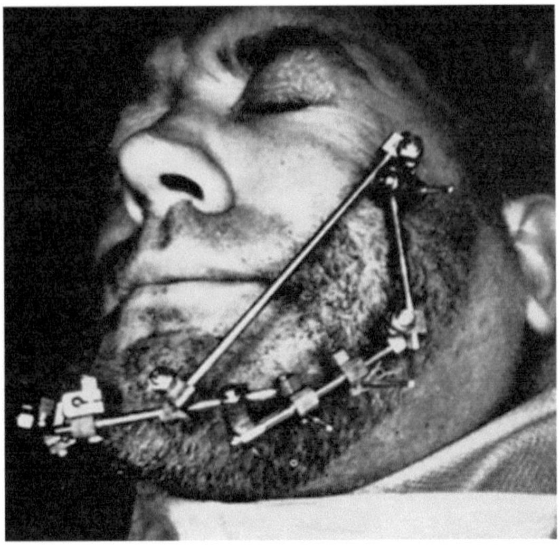

**Fig. 15.2** External fixation with malar pins

mandibular fixation methods for immobilizing the mandible when teeth are inadequate for intermaxillary fixation. The advantages of these two methods are also compared to other approaches to mandible immobilization such as the Barton bandage and skeletal fixation (Fig. 15.1). With the Barton bandage, the bandage can loosen or move, limiting its effectiveness in immobilization. Skeletal fixation connects the fracture appliance to the skeleton by single malar pins bilaterally, but the pins can be insufficient in resisting mandibular forces (Fig. 15.2).

The external craniomandibular fixation method can be utilized when dentition is inadequate for intermaxillary fixation. If the patient is edentulous, a denture or Gunning splint can be used to maintain occlusion. The external craniomandibular fixation method uses FracSure extension rods that extend from a plaster headcap and attach to the mandible for fracture fixation. If the patient has an anterior mandible symphysis fracture, the FracSure rods can connect to a Kirschner wire or Steinmann pin.

As first described by Thoma in 1943, internal maxillomandibular fixation may be used for patients with complete upper dentures who have at least mandibular anterior teeth but can be adapted for completely edentulous patients as well. The primary advantage of internal fixation is that there is no need for a headcap or external appliance, allowing the patient to return to normal day-to-day activities sooner.

Two methods for internal fixation were described. The first requires the upper denture in place and application of arch wires to the mandibular anterior teeth. Then, wires are inserted through the piriform aperture and attached to the mandibular arch wire. Mandibular partial dentures may be worn as well but are not necessary.

The second method requires the application of circumferential wires to secure a mandibular Gunning splint. The ends of the circumferential wires are then attached to wires inserted through the margins of the piriform aperture. For completely edentulous patients, a Gunning splint to the upper and lower jaw may be fabricated, or alternatively the patients' upper and lower dentures may be used as a substitute.

It is important to contextualize Dr. Thoma's work in his paper "New Methods for the Immobilization of the mandible" with a brief review of the history of mandible fracture management to understand the importance of his contributions at the time. As early as thirty centuries BC in the Egyptian text the Smith Papyrus, there is documentation of treatment of facial fractures [1]. Hippocrates had described a method for immobilizing a fractured mandible with strips of leather glued to the skin for direct traction along with manual reduction and intraoral immobilization by tying gold or linen threads around adjacent teeth [1]. Different variations of external bandages and simple ligatures around teeth for mandible fracture immobilization and fixation remained the classical standard for fracture management for centuries following. However, a core issue with this approach was the instability of the fracture segments. In the eighteenth century, Pierre Fauchard published *Traité de chirurgie dentaire* outlining a systematic approach to dentistry and denture construction, which served as a basis for others to push forward innovations with dental prostheses that could better stabilize a mandible in fracture management [2].

The nineteenth and twentieth centuries then saw many refinements and advances in techniques for splint design, external fixation, and wire fixation aided by the discovery of anesthesia by Horace Wells in 1844 [3]. This included the Gunning splint developed by Thomas Gunning in 1866, a one-piece splint which could be modified for patients with edentulous jaws. The original splints were made from a single piece of vulcanite rubber with a space placed anteriorly to allow for nutrition. Screws were used to fixate the splint to the occlusal surfaces of teeth, the hard palate, or the mandible [4]. It was Thoma who first reported to stabilize such splints with wire passed through the piriform aperture [2, 5]. He also detailed how a denture could be used as a substitute in edentulous cases (Fig. 15.3).

Gilmer rediscovered intermaxillary fixation in 1887, a technique which had not been used for centuries, which involved the use of wire to ligate teeth in the upper and lower jaws to one another in order to immobilize the mandible [2]. Gilmer later modified the technique further to involve the use of an arch bar which followed the outer contour of the dental arch. His original method was later improved upon by Oliver (1910) and Ivy (1922) and later described by Thoma as part of the technique used for internal maxillomandibular fixation with wires passed through the margin of the piriform aperture holding the maxillary denture in place [2, 5] (Fig. 15.4a, b).

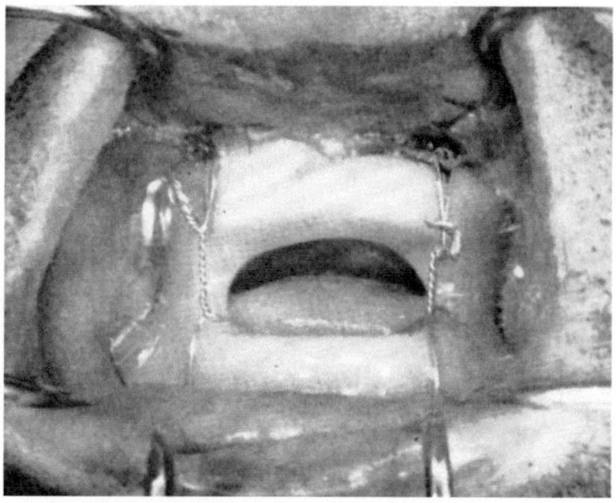

**Fig. 15.3** Acrylic splint wired to mandible and secured by wires passed through margin of piriform aperture

In 1897, Clayton Parkhill pushed forward the evolution of external fixation in the United States by attaching bone "clamps" to fractured bone segments [6]. Later the use of Kirschner wires for mandible fracture treatment was described in 1932, where pins were inserted transcutaneously into the bone segments for fracture fixation after the establishment of occlusion [3]. Particular impetus for advances in technique and technology for external and internal fixation for mandibular fracture treatment then came during World War II [2].

In his 1948 paper "New Methods for Immobilization of the Mandible," Thoma discussed a method of external fixation that used a plaster headcap and FracSure extension rods to improve fracture stability by better withstanding masticatory forces on the fractures in comparison to only using malar implants for external fixation (Fig. 15.5a, b) [5]. While there was some success with external fixation using pins during his time, Thoma felt his method improved fracture stability particularly where other techniques of pin fixation were insufficient for cases of mandible fractures in edentulous patients [7]. He also reviewed how his approach to external fixation could be adapted to incorporate Gunning splints and Kirschner wires if required for management of an edentulous patient.

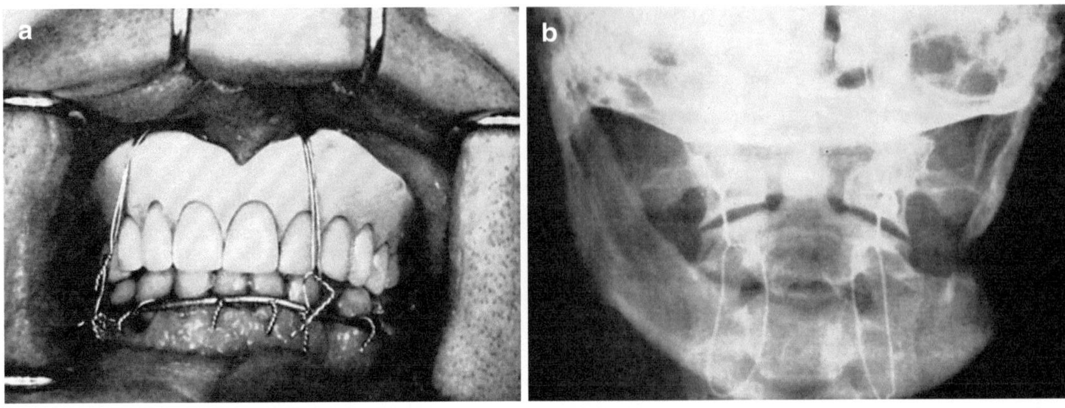

**Fig. 15.4** (**a**) Internal maxillomandibular fixation with wires passed through piriform aperture and wired to mandibular arch wire with upper denture in place. (**b**) Anteroposterior view X-ray demonstrating splint supported by mandibular circumferential wires and wires through the margin of the piriform aperture

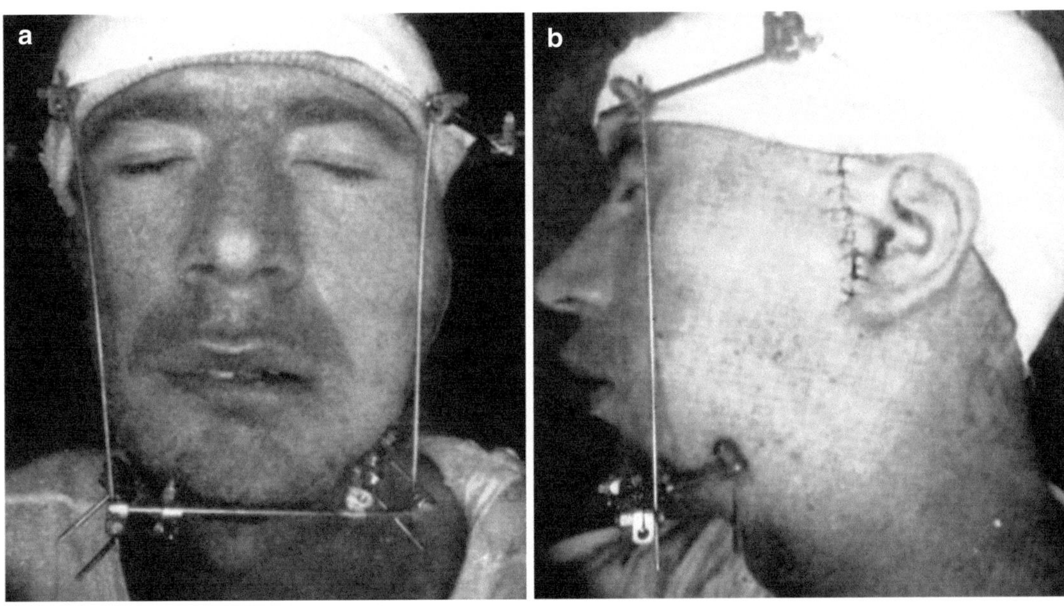

**Fig. 15.5** (**a**, **b**) External fixation with plaster cap and FracSure extension rods. With option of including Gunning splint for edentulous patients

Compression plate osteosynthesis was not applied to maxillofacial fractures until Hans Luhr introduced the concept in 1968 [8]. With advancements in osteosynthesis and rigid internal fixation with plating, the utility of external fixation for mandible fractures today is limited to particular indications including cases of emergent management of complex multi-fragment facial trauma, defects where atraumatic soft tissue preservation is priority, or pathological fractures [9]. However during his time, Thoma pushed forward techniques in external fixation that enhanced stability of mandible fractures before these future discoveries in mandible immobilization and treatment were made.

The editors of this book chose a number of surgeons whose techniques or teachings have helped move the specialty of oral and maxillofacial surgery forward. The authors of this chapter have been honored to be asked to write about this amazing individual who in addition to the paper he published in 1948 in the Triple "O" Journal entitled "New Methods for the Immobilization of the Mandible" published many articles and books: *Oral Anesthesia*, *Oral Abscesses*, *Oral Roentgenology*, *Teeth, Diet and Health*, *Clinical Pathology of the Jaws*, *Oral Diagnosis*, *Oral Pathology*, and *Oral Surgery*. Many of these books were published as multiple editions.

In addition to the books and articles, he advanced the field of oral surgery and oral pathology. He was the founding editor of the *Journal of Oral Surgery*, *Oral Medicine* and *Oral Pathology*. He enjoyed appointments as a professor at Harvard School of Dental Medicine, Boston University Graduate School of Dentistry, and the University of Pennsylvania Graduate School of Medicine. He was awarded fellowships in several organizations and honorary societies.

Kurt Thoma was born in Basel Switzerland in 1883, he attended the Institute of Technology where he was studying architecture. In 1908, he emigrated to Boston to attend the Harvard School of Dental Medicine where he graduated cum laude in 1911. He subsequently returned to Switzerland to study the use of procaine in dental anesthesia. He returned to Boston to teach the use of procaine as a dental anesthetic. He knew of the use of procaine when he experienced dental pain and he had a tooth extraction with minimal discomfort. After his period of learning in Switzerland, he returned to become an assistant in anesthesia at Harvard.

The next year he was appointed an assistant in anatomy. Dr. Thoma also studied embryology which led to his interest in oral pathology; he was a founding member of the American Academy of Oral Pathology. He wrote the first of his eight books with the publication of *Oral Anesthesiology* in 1914. This was followed by *Oral Abscesses* in 1916 and *Oral Roentgenology* in 1917.

He married Louise Bird in 1912 and had a son and daughter. One might wonder what Dr. Thoma did this in his "spare time." He designed his home, maintained a professional garden, was an accomplished equestrian, and an avid hunter and fisherman. He was a friend of some of the great names in medicine: Drs. Frank Lahey, Delbert Jackson, Lewis Hill, Delos Bristol, Homer Sowles, and Victor Carpenter. He maintained a full private practice and multiple hospital appointments.

He accomplished much in his lifetime while he maintained active hospital appointments and an active private practice. He authored Teeth, Diet and Health in 1923, *Clinical Pathology of the Jaws* 1925, *Oral Diagnosis and Treatment Planning* 1936, *Oral Pathology* 1941, with many following editions, and *Oral Surgery* 1948 with many following editions.

His influence in OMFS was eclipsed by his contributions to oral pathology: founder of the American Board of Oral Pathology, Editor of Oral Surgery, Oral Medicine and Oral Pathology from 1948 to 1970, Professor of Oral Surgery at Boston University Goldman School of Dental Medicine, Professor of Oral Pathology and Oral Surgery at Harvard School of Dental Medicine, and Professor of Oral Surgery at Pennsylvania School of Dental Medicine. There were many awards bestowed on Dr. Thoma: Royal College of Surgeons Edinburgh and England, Jarvie Award, Alfred Fones Medal, Pierre Fauchard Medal, and Tomes Lectureship of the Royal College of Surgeons.

Dr. Thoma died on June 5, 1972; his life was full of firsts and he demonstrated what a well-trained dentist and oral surgeon can accomplish. There are very few who can surpass his accomplishments across a broad spectrum. The authors would like to borrow a quote from Daniel J. Hollands' eulogy: "Historically, in every specialty there have been a handful of strong determined, resourceful men who set the pace, defined the goals, defended the boundaries and undaunted by obstacles, thus made it infinitely easier for succeeding generations to follow." Kurt H. Thoma has long been recognized as the father of oral pathology, the defender of oral surgery, and the great teacher of oral medicine. He raised the standards, developed surgical techniques, and encouraged several generations of oral surgeons to a high level of professional stature. Those who train students and trainees aspire to a similar level of teaching for future generations of oral and maxillofacial surgeons. Dr. Thoma is one of the greats and would be pleased by what his legacy has brought.

## References


1. Dingman R, Natvig P. Surgery of facial fractures. 1st ed. Philadelphia, PA: W. B. Saunders Company; 1964. p. 11–42.
2. Rowe NL. The history of the treatment of maxillo-facial trauma. Ann R Coll Surg Engl. 1971;49(5):329–49. https://www.ncbi.nlm.nih.gov/pmc/articles/PMC2388034/?tool=pmcentrez&report=abstract
3. Mukerji R, Mukerji G, McGurk M. Mandibular fractures: historical perspective. Br J Oral Maxillofac Surg. 2006;44(3):222–8. https://doi.org/10.1016/j.bjoms.2005.06.023.
4. Gunning TB. Treatment of fracture of the lower jaw by interdental splints. Am J Dent Sci. 1868;2(3):106–20.
5. Thoma KH. New methods for immobilization of the mandible. Oral Surg Oral Med Oral Pathol Oral Radiol Endod. 2005;100(2):S5–S10. https://doi.org/10.1016/j.tripleo.2005.05.004.
6. Parkhill C. A new apparatus for the fixation of bones after resection and in fractures with a tendency to displacement: with report of cases. Clin Orthop Relat Res. 1983;180:3–6. https://journals.lww.com/clinorthop/Abstract/1983/11000/A_New_Apparatus_for_the_Fixation_of_Bones_after.2.aspx
7. Rushton MA, Walker FA. Mandibular fractures treated by pin fixation: twenty-one cases. Am J Orthodontics Oral Surg. 1942;28(5):B307–15. https://doi.org/10.1016/S0096-6347(42)90507-6.
8. Luhr HG. Zur stabilen Osteosynthese bei Unterkieferfrakturen [On the stable osteosynthesis in mandibular fractures]. Dtsch Zahnarztl Z. 1968;23(7):754. German. PMID: 5242894.
9. Cornelius CP, Augustin JB, Sailer LK. External pin fixation for stabilization of the mandible—comeback of a method: historical review and first experiences with the 'mandible external fixator'. Oral Maxillofac Surg. 2004;13:1–14. https://doi.org/10.1007/s10006-008-0142-4.

# Three-Dimensional Approach to Analysis and Treatment of Hemifacial Microsomia [1]

16

Daniel P. Caruso, Cameron C. Lee, and Zachary S. Peacock

**Abstract**

In Dr. Leonard Kaban's 1981 paper entitled, "Three-Dimensional Approach to Analysis and Treatment of Hemifacial Microsomia" (Kaban et al., Cleft Palate J. 18:90–99, 1981), the authors challenged the single radiograph assessment paradigm. The study published in the *Cleft Palate Journal* proposed a three-dimensional analysis utilizing sagittal, anteroposterior, and submental X-ray views to fully classify the defect utilizing the authors' experiences with a cohort of 40 patients with hemifacial microsomia (Fig. 16.1).

The Kaban study was the first to describe hemifacial microsomia in more than one dimension in the era before readily available computed tomography (CT). Prior to this, the lateral cephalogram was used commonly to describe the deformity in one plane. The report changed the assessment of hemifacial microsomia and improved the understanding of the primary and secondary deformity. The assessment remains important when planning treatment of hemifacial microsomia despite CT long becoming the standard of care in craniomaxillofacial surgery.

**Keywords**

Hemifacial microsomia · Three-dimensional · Mandibular growth · Craniofacial anomaly

## Background of the Study

Hemifacial microsomia can be grouped into three categories based on severity of the mandibular anomaly: (I) hypoplasia of the mandible and temporomandibular joint (TMJ); (II) hypoplastic and abnormally shaped ramus with an underdeveloped and medially displaced TMJ; and (III) absent ramus and glenoid fossa [2]. Other features of this deformity (e.g., ear deformities, facial nerve dysfunction, and soft tissue deficiencies) do not always correlate with the severity of underlying skeletal deformity. Roughly 20–30% of patients have bilateral abnormalities, with one side usually more affected. Often the less severe side may have a mild external ear abnormality or a preauricular skin tag with more normal underlying skeleton.

D. P. Caruso · Z. S. Peacock (✉)
Department of Oral and Maxillofacial Surgery, Harvard School of Dental Medicine, Boston, MA, USA

Division of Oral and Maxillofacial Surgery, Massachusetts General Hospital, Boston, MA, USA
e-mail: dpcaruso@partners.org; zpeacock@partners.org

C. C. Lee
Department of Oral and Maxillofacial Surgery, Harvard School of Dental Medicine, Boston, MA, USA

Division of Oral and Maxillofacial Surgery, Massachusetts General Hospital, Boston, MA, USA

University of Maryland, College Park, MD, USA
e-mail: clee48@partners.org



S. R. Aziz, M. D. Turner (eds.), *Classic Papers and Pioneers in Maxillofacial and Oral Surgery*,
https://doi.org/10.1007/978-3-031-63246-4_16

Dr. Kaban and coauthors described hemifacial microsomia within the context of facial growth and the secondary effects of the deformity. The mandibular deformity was hypothesized to be the earliest skeletal manifestation and therefore results in a secondary distortion of the midface. The abnormal mandibular growth has been defined as the "keystone" feature. During normal growth and development, the mandibular ramus lengthens and moves posteriorly. The lengthening occurs as a result of bone deposition on the posterior–inferior surface of the ramus and bony resorption on the anterior surface. Resorption of the anterior ramus subsequently leads to elongation of the mandibular body. Similarly, mandibular width increases with bone deposition on the lateral surface and resorption of the medial surface. Concurrently, the maxilla grows in an inferior and anterior direction due to bone resorption of the superior nasal surface and deposition on the palatal surface.

In hemifacial microsomia, the unilateral mandibular growth impairment results in deviation of the mandibular dental midline and symphysis toward the affected side. In the transverse plane, lack of remodeling results in a narrow mandibular body and medially displaced ramus. The shortened mandible and superiorly tilted occlusal plane on the affected side restricts downward growth of the maxilla and inhibits the usual bony separation between the maxillary alveolus, piriform, and orbit. In some cases, the zygoma may also be hypoplastic.

## Methods of the Study

The proposed three-dimensional (3D) analysis included the sagittal, frontal, and transverse planes via panoramic, lateral cephalometric, anteroposterior (AP) cephalometric, and submental radiographic views (Fig. 16.1).

### Sagittal Plane

The panoramic radiograph reveals the shape of the TMJs and rami. The ramus-condylar unit heights can be measured to assess the morphologic discrepancy between sides. The lateral cephalometric analysis shows the difference in ramus height, the overlying asymmetry, and the maxilla relative to the mandible.

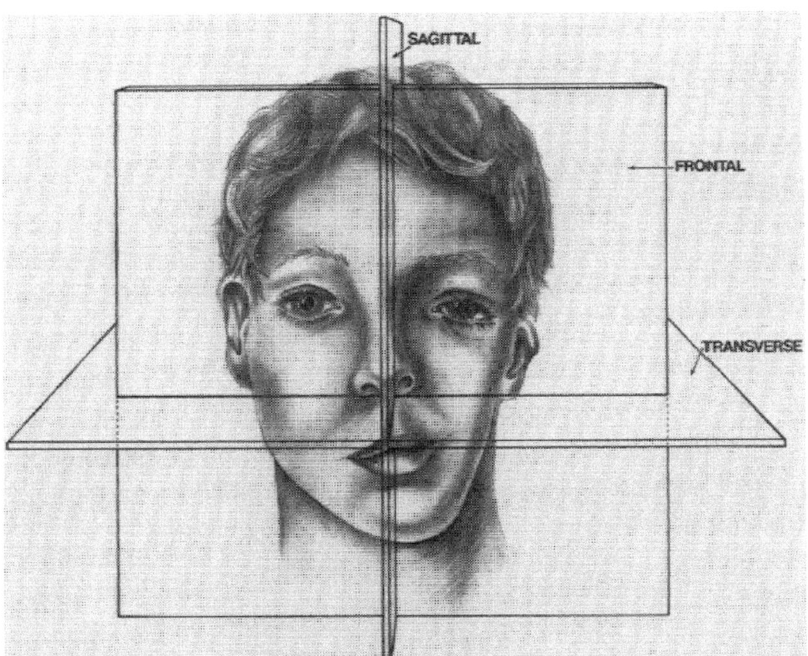


**Fig. 16.1** Drawing from the original manuscript [1] depicting the three planes to describe the deformity of hemifacial microsomia (sagittal, frontal, and transverse). (Used with permission from American Cleft Palate Association)

## Frontal Plane

The AP cephalometric radiograph provides a different view of the asymmetric rami and allows visualization of the pyriform aperture and orbits. A vertical midline reference plane can be created to assess the degree of mandibular dental/skeletal midline deviation, medial displacement of the ramus and glenoid fossa, and obliquity of occlusal plane.

## Transverse Plane

The submental vertex radiograph demonstrates the shape/width of the mandibular arch, medial/anterior displacement of the TMJs, and zygomatic asymmetry.

# Application of Study Concepts

The authors showcased the application of their proposed 3D analysis and highlight their thought process by reviewing several cases, one for each mandible type of hemifacial microsomia.

## Type I

The type I mandible was described as deficiency in ramus height, tilting of the pyriform, deviation of the mandibular skeletal midline, and decreased mandibular width. Therefore, correction entailed left ramus elongation with a compensatory contralateral osteotomy. The mandible was rotated, and a posterior segmental osteotomy was performed to widen the arch and establish stable occlusion.

## Type II (Less Severe)

The authors described the less severe type II mandible (later described as Kaban IIa) as follows: short ramus height, underdeveloped TMJ, mandibular skeletal/dental midline deviation, medially displaced ramus, and anteromedially displaced TMJ. Correction involved bilateral ramus osteotomies with an interpositional graft on the affected side to elongate the ramus and enhance the lateral contour at the angle. The more normal side was elongated using a sliding oblique osteotomy. The mandible was rotated, and an open bite was maintained in the premolar segment to allow for orthodontic widening of the arch.

## Type II (More Severe)

The more severe type II mandible (later referred to as Kaban IIb) has a severely displaced and shortened ramus. Correction was accomplished by excising a portion of the abnormal ramus and constructing the ramus-condyle unit with autogenous grafts (e.g., costochondral rib graft). A compensatory osteotomy was performed on the more normal side to facilitate midline correction.

## Type III

The most severe deformity (type III) was described as an absent ramus and TMJ with a medially displaced mandible. A costochondral graft was used to create a ramus-condylar unit which was positioned as lateral as possible. In the case example, the authors also constructed a zygomatic arch.

# Study Discussion

Management of hemifacial microsomia requires understanding of the mandibular growth pattern and overall deformity progression. Dr. Kaban and his coauthors argued for the need to change perspective from the paradigm of one-dimensional treatment of end stage defects to three-dimensional analysis with intervention during growth. The rationale was that early intervention may unlock growth on the affected side and prevent secondary distortion of the maxilla, pyriform rim, and orbits.

The other impact of viewing all three dimensions is the resultant change in operative approach. Earlier corrections involved only lengthening the affected ramus. With this "one-dimensional" treatment, patients would have limited function and stability because the ramus-condyle unit was not corrected in the frontal plane. Treatment planning in three dimensions allows for more symmetric and physiologic jaw function.

## Summary

"Three-Dimensional Approach to Analysis and Treatment of Hemifacial Microsomia" [1] is Dr. Kaban's earliest publication on the topic of hemifacial microsomia. He would go on to publish 12 original articles regarding diagnosis and management of this congenital deformity and is widely considered a leading expert on the condition. In 1969, Dr. Samuel Pruzansky introduced the classification system for the mandibular defect in patients with hemifacial microsomia [2]. Dr. Kaban added a modification to this classification system in his 1988 paper entitled, "Surgical Correction of Hemifacial Microsomia in the Growing Child" [3]. He separated type II into type IIA or type IIB, with the latter consisting of a markedly abnormal ramus-condylar unit located anteromedially and having no articulation with the temporal bone. The Kaban modification of the Pruzansky classification remains the standard for describing the mandibular defect.

Dr. Kaban's subsequent work characterized the progressive nature of hemifacial microsomia. He advocated for early intervention to lengthen the mandible in the mixed dentition to prevent secondary distortion of the midface. In one of his most recent papers on the subject, "Mandibular Asymmetry and the Fourth Dimension" [4], Dr. Kaban synthesizes his greater than 30 years of experience and collaboration with Dr. Joseph Murray and Dr. John Mulliken to underscore the importance of time in the assessment and treatment of congenital and acquired facial deformities.

## Biography

Dr. Kaban was born and raised in New York City. He attended Queens College, City University of New York and graduated in 1966. He received a full Regents Scholarship to pursue either a medical degree or dental degree within the state of New York. However, he was recruited to Harvard School of Dental Medicine (HSDM) by the dean, Dr. Howard Oaks. After a discussion with his uncle who was a physician, he made the difficult decision to leave New York and attend Harvard in hopes of broadening his horizons and challenging himself in a new environment.

During his second year at HSDM, he discovered a passion for pediatrics while shadowing in the craniofacial clinic at Boston Children's Hospital (BCH). In 1969, he graduated at the top of his class and chose to complete a residency in oral and maxillofacial surgery (OMS) at Massachusetts General Hospital (MGH). When Dr. Kaban started residency, there were no dual-degree programs. Dr. Walter Guralnick, Chief of the OMS Department at MGH, established the first combined MD pathway, which was officially approved in 1972. Dr. Kaban was one of the first residents to take advantage of this opportunity, and after completing his residency in 1972, he went on to obtain his MD from Harvard Medical School in 1974.

After residency, he was hired as the head of the newly founded oral surgery division at Brigham and Women's Hospital (BWH) and BCH, becoming the first full time oral and maxillofacial surgeon to be employed at both institutions. Under the mentorship of Dr. Joseph Murray, Chief of Plastic and Oral Surgery, Dr.

Kaban developed a successful practice. After only 6 months, MGH began to send OMS residents to train with Dr. Kaban.

Dr. Kaban's passion for research blossomed during his years at BCH. Dr. Murray fostered a culture of academic productivity and believed that all surgeons should be involved in research. It was with this mentality that the team of Murray, John B. Mulliken, Kaban, and Joseph Upton published over 70 studies between 1974 and 1985. The skills and discipline that Dr. Kaban learned during this period were carried forward to his own training programs in the future.

In 1985, Dr. Kaban accepted the position of Professor and Chairman of the Department of OMS at the University of California, San Francisco (UCSF). He also served as the Associate Dean for Hospital Relations at the UCSF School of Dentistry. One of his biggest accomplishments during this time was the establishment of the dual-degree program at UCSF. He remained in California until 1994 when he received an opportunity to return to Boston. Dr. Bruce Donoff had become the Dean of HSDM, thus vacating the position of Chief of the OMS Department at MGH. In doing so, he became the Walter C. Guralnick Professor and Chairman for the Department of OMFS at HSDM.

As Chief at MGH, Dr. Kaban strove to inspire the same culture of academic productivity as his mentor, Dr. Murray. He promptly established a thematic research program, thus making research inseparable from the clinical duties and patient care of all attending faculty members. As part of this endeavor, he founded the Skeletal Biology Research Center to study the molecular basis of bone healing in distraction osteogenesis in large animal models. As an area of particular interest, Dr. Kaban has published nearly 40 articles on distraction osteogenesis and recently won the Daniel Laskin Award for best paper in the *Journal of Oral and Maxillofacial Surgery* for his 2018 manuscript entitled, "Long Term Effects of Distraction Osteogenesis of the Mandible" [5].

Other areas of research that thrived under Dr. Kaban's tenure include tissue engineering and giant cell tumors. With research incorporated seamlessly into clinical practice at MGH, the department produced 559 publications and converted 74% of abstracts to publications between the years 2000 and 2012. Dr. Kaban has won several research awards including the American Association of Oral and Maxillofacial Surgeons (AAOMS) Award for Excellence in Clinical Research (2017) and the Norton M. Ross Award for Excellence in Clinical Research from the American Dental Association.

Education is another key part of Dr. Kaban's legacy. Since he began working with trainees in 1974, he has trained and mentored more than 100 residents and fellows. In keeping with his goal of producing clinician-scientists, he established the MGH Fellowship in Research and Pediatric OMS. The fellowship was 50% clinical and 50% research oriented with a focus on minimally invasive surgery and distraction osteogenesis. In honor of Dr. Kaban and his commitment to research, patient care, and education, the Leonard B. Kaban, DMD, MD Chair in Pediatric Oral and Maxillofacial Surgery at BCH was established, with Dr. Bonnie Padwa as the first incumbent.

Dr. Kaban stepped down as the Chief of OMS in 2015 after leading the MGH OMS Department for 21 years. Throughout his career he has made countless contributions to the specialty of OMS and has proven himself as a true pioneer in the field. He has published broadly about many subjects but is particularly well known for his impact within pediatric surgery and craniofacial deformities. He has authored over 300 scientific manuscripts and co-authored 8 textbooks including the definitive text for pediatrics, entitled *Pediatric Oral and Maxillofacial Surgery*. His legacy will be as an outstanding clinician, researcher, and innovator, a combination rarely seen with such vigor (Fig. 16.2).

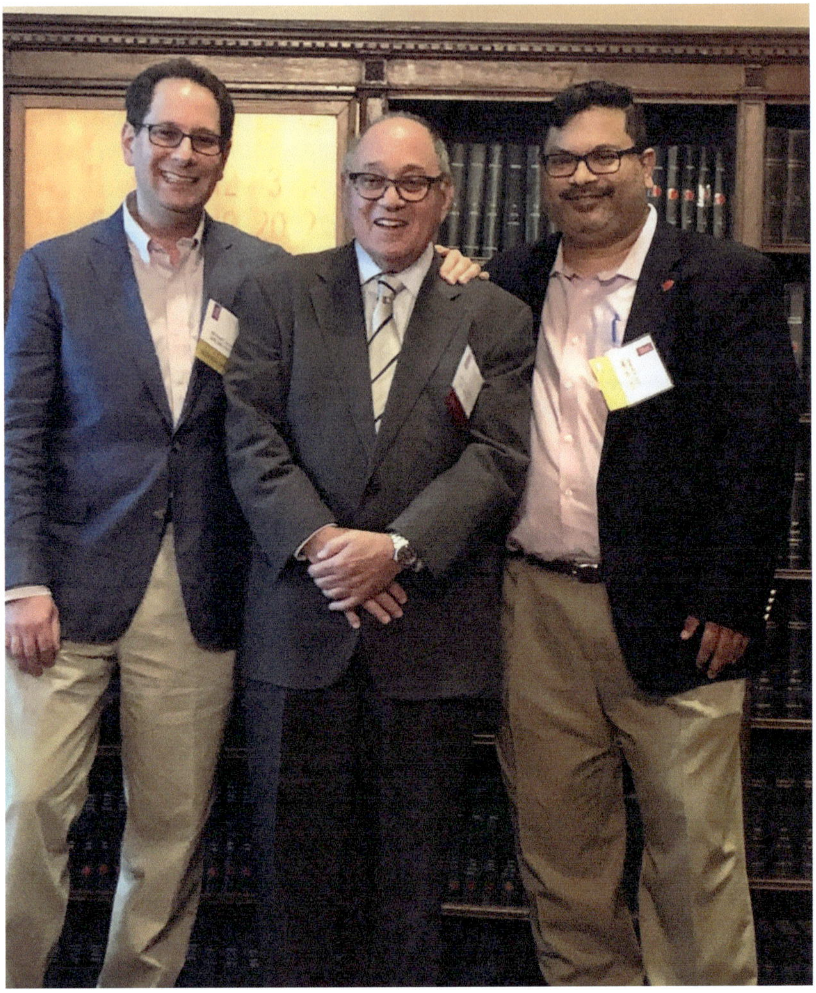

**Fig. 16.2** From left to right: Drs Michael Turner, Leonard Kaban, and Shahid Aziz circa 2018 New York Academy of Medicine Annual Oral and Maxillofacial Surgery Residents' night

## References


1. Kaban LB, Mulliken JB, Murray JE. Three-dimensional approach to analysis and treatment of hemifacial microsomia. Cleft Palate J. 1981;18(2):90–9.
2. Pruzansky S. Not all dwarfed mandibles are alike. Birth Defects. 1969;4:120.
3. Kaban LB, Padwa BL, Mulliken JB. Surgical correction of mandibular hypoplasia in hemifacial microsomia: the case for treatment in early childhood. J Oral Maxillofac Surg. 1998;56(5):628–38. https://doi.org/10.1016/s0278-2391(98)90465-7.
4. Kaban LB. Mandibular asymmetry and the fourth dimension. J Craniofac Surg. 2009;20(Suppl 1):622–31. https://doi.org/10.1097/SCS.0b013e318195249c.
5. Peacock ZS, Salcines A, Troulis MJ, Kaban LB. Long-term effects of distraction osteogenesis of the mandible. J Oral Maxillofac Surg. 2018;76(7):1512–23. https://doi.org/10.1016/j.joms.2017.12.034.

# 17 The Combined Oral Surgery-MD Program: The Harvard Plan. J Oral Surg. 1973 Apr; 31(4):271–6. PMID: 4510650

Leonard B. Kaban and David A. Keith

**Abstract**

Dr. Walter Guralnick played a significant role in the evolution of the specialty of Oral and Maxillofacial Surgery in the United States: he was a surgeon, researcher, academic, and leader. However, perhaps his greatest accomplishment was development of the dual-degree oral and maxillofacial surgery (OMS)-MD program. Within this program, an OMS resident would receive the required oral and maxillofacial surgery and anesthesia training, as well as general surgery training and most importantly the opportunity to complete medical school. Obtaining the doctor of medicine degree by the oral and maxillofacial surgeon ensured that the specialty would maintain an equal footing among other surgical specialties. This was perhaps Guralnick's most important legacy.

**Keywords**

Oral & Maxillofacial surgery · Guralnick · Surgical education · Massachusetts General Hospital · Harvard School of Dental Medicine · Harvard Medical School

L. B. Kaban (✉) · D. A. Keith
Department of Oral and Maxillofacial Surgery, Massachusetts General Hospital, Harvard School of Dental Medicine, Boston, MA, USA
e-mail: kaban.leonard@mgh.harvard.edu; lkaban@partners.org; DKEITH@mgh.harvard.edu

## Introduction

Many surgeons receive accolades for their surgical innovations, for example, new operations or modifications of existing operations that change practice and improve patients' lives. Others excel in clinical or basic research; their results and writings improve surgical knowledge and advance the scope of a surgical specialty. Some are inspiring clinical teachers, thereby safeguarding and enhancing the competence of the next generation of surgeons. Finally, surgeons may contribute to the realm of service to the community, hospital, specialty, and/or humanitarian organizations. Dr. Walter C. Guralnick who was Professor and Chief of the Department of Oral and Maxillofacial Surgery (OMFS) at Massachusetts General Hospital (MGH) and Harvard School of Dental Medicine (HSDM) from 1967 to 1983 was active in all these areas, as his biography below will show. However, his most important and influential legacy is probably demonstrated by this publication in the *Journal of Oral Surgery* (JOS), as it was then called, in 1973: **Guralnick WC. The combined oral surgery-MD program: the Harvard plan. J Oral Surg. 1973 Apr;31(4):271–6. PMID: 4510650** [1].



S. R. Aziz, M. D. Turner (eds.), *Classic Papers and Pioneers in Maxillofacial and Oral Surgery*,
https://doi.org/10.1007/978-3-031-63246-4_17

## Summary of Article

Guralnick, in the introduction to the paper, articulates that he understood the resistance to the changes he was proposing in oral surgery (OS) education and the accusations that would be leveled at him in this process: "A major curricular change cannot be made without considerable trauma to the group affected by it. Being aware of this, we certainly would not have instituted a new oral surgical training program were we not convinced that there was a serious need of innovation." He goes on to explain that after 30 years in clinical practice and educating students and residents, he concluded that there was an educational deficit in OS residency programs that consisted of: "…insufficient general medical and surgical background…" which would be "corrected best by obtaining a medical degree and general surgery" training in addition to the OS experience. Guralnick also indicated that his commitment to training "doubly-qualified" surgeons was "not motivated by personal frustration, pique, vanity, or irresponsibility" and that his "clinical activity as an oral surgeon has been unfettered, throughout my career, by self-seeking reasons of colleagues in medicine or dentistry."

Finally, Guralnick appreciated that the MD degree and general surgery training would improve the respect and stature of OSs within the hospital, university, and general medical community. He was also one of the first OS chiefs in the United States to appreciate and implement the "full-time" faculty model in the specialty. These two changes or improvements in OS training programs have had long-term effects on the scope of practice of oral and maxillofacial surgery (OMS) and the specialty's place in academic medical centers and hospitals. In 2018, the American College of Surgeons (ACS) recognized the credentials of dual-degree oral and maxillofacial surgeons (OMS) for fellowship and subsequently approved fellowship for single-degree OMSs.

In this article, Guralnick describes oral surgery's long-term concern with education, training, and improvement in standards of care. This began in 1918 with the American Society of Exodontists and Oral Surgeons and extended through several name iterations to American Society of Oral Surgeons (and ultimately, years after this article was published, to the American Association of Oral and Maxillofacial Surgeons, AAOMS). Another milestone was the establishment of the American Board of Oral Surgery in 1946 and subsequently, the name-change to American Board of Oral and Maxillofacial Surgery (ABOMS). Modifications and advances in the quality of OMS education and expansion of continuing education improved standards and quality of practice. In the article, Guralnick relates that a series of conferences held by the society resulted in the publication of: *The Essentials of an Advanced Education Program in Oral Surgery* in 1959. This served as a guide to achieve a "high level of consistency in the education offered by accredited training programs and to ensure that residents who complete these programs acquire a predictable level of competence." Dr. Guralnick was Chairman of the AAOMS Committee on Residency Education and Training (1973–1980) and during his tenure, the Oral and Maxillofacial Surgery In-training Examination (OMSITE) was developed and implemented. The examination has been given yearly since 1977 and has served as a benchmark for Program Directors, Department Chiefs, and faculty to evaluate their residents and training programs [2].

Guralnick relates the observations of nationally prominent oral surgeons who describe difficulties for the specialty because of a lack of an MD degree. James Hayward, editor-in-chief of the JOS decried "the barriers due to union prejudice" and predicted that future progress in oral surgery education would require the complex cooperation/collaboration of the professions of dentistry and medicine as well as hospitals [3]. In 1968, Dr. Robert Shira (General in the Army, Head of the Army Dental Corps, and editor-in-chief of the journal *Oral Surgery, Oral Medicine and Oral Pathology*), in his Chalmers Lyons Lecture, noted that OS must be vigilant in maintaining high standards and consistency in our training programs and that the future of the specialty depends on the education and training we provide for our residents [4]. Shira and Guralnick were concerned about the future of OS as a specialty and OS education. They noted problems that existed because of the lack of an MD degree, including difficulties with the Joint Commission on Hospital Accreditation and the American Medical Association regarding DDS surgeons encroaching on the practice of medicine. They also described exclusion from Medicare and Federal Employees Health Plans and lack of payment for OSs by various private insurance companies which limited reimbursement only to physicians. "There is no doubt that limitations on the scope of oral surgery practice exist in some hospitals including instances of harassment, limitation of privileges, seizure of cases, adverse rulings and frank antagonism." Both Shira and Guralnick considered the advantages and disadvantages of adding an MD degree to OS training [1, 4].

It should be noted that a group of OSs personally pursued the MD degree and general surgery training after World War II (WWII) through the 1960s. These pioneers are identified in the publication by Perrott and Kaban: History of dual-degree oral and maxillofacial surgery training in the United States in the *Journal of Oral and Maxillofacial Surgery* [5]. Guralnick, in the 1973 paper, identifies the benefits of double-degree training, including a broader educational background, more surgical experience, a better profile within medical centers, hospitals, and hospital operating rooms to correspond with the increasing scope of OMS practice beginning after WWII. Guralnick, paraphrasing Shira's address, also pointed out that there would be two possible disadvantages of dual-degree training: (1) "Specialized oral surgery training [component] might be impaired by shortening its length" and (2) "Expense and time involved would be overwhelming and discourage potential applicants and loss of residents to other specialties" [1, 4].

Guralnick recognized certain opportunities that were occurring in the late 1960s and early 1970s with changing medical school curricula. Some schools were offering the MD degree in 3 years and in other medical schools, the fourth year was entirely elective. An opportunity available at Harvard School of Dental Medicine (HSDM) and a few other dental schools was that dental students spent the first 2 years in their respective medical school's curriculum. Therefore, the only thing they were missing for the MD degree was the principal clinical year experience. With this realization, Guralnick was able to formulate a 5-year program for Harvard students that would provide the required number of months of OS, the MD degree, and 18 months of general surgery training. He observed that this "was not prohibitively longer than many oral surgery programs" (some were going to 4 years with increasing off service rotations) and therefore "Shira's objections are no longer valid." Meetings with the Deans of HSDM and Harvard Medical School (HMS) and the Chiefs of General and Plastic Surgery at MGH produced support for the MD degree and general surgery core training for OS residents. The concern that applicants would use the program as a "back door" to an MD degree was addressed by starting the program with 12 continuous months of OS internship. This experience would acquaint residents with the full breadth and scope of OS and firmly bolster their commitment to the specialty. In addition, the MD degree was awarded at the end of the third year of the program. This sequence would minimize the risk of loss of residents to other specialties.

## Description of the Combined MGH Harvard-MD Oral Surgery Program Approved in 1970

The sequence of the Harvard Program is shown in Table 17.1 [1, 5].

[The first trainee to enroll in the program as written and approved was John PW Kelly who started as an OS intern in 1971 and graduated in 1976. R. Bruce Donoff, Steven Roser, Edward Seldin, and Leonard Kaban who were, at the time, either junior or senior residents in the 3-year hospital-based program were accepted to HMS for the MD degree and the MGH for a year of general surgery. They received 1 additional year of general surgery credit for their 3-month general surgery rotation plus the 2 years of OS training. They completed their training in 1973 (Roser and Seldin) and 1974 (Donoff and Kaban). Several other residents (Harry Schwartz and Thomas Albert) were accepted for a double-

**Table 17.1** The Harvard Program

| |
|---|
| Year 1: Oral Surgery Internship, 12 months |
| Year 2: Principal clinical year at Harvard Medical School |
| Year 3: Assistant Resident Oral Surgery 6 months; Intern in General Surgery 6 months; MD degree awarded |
| Year 4: Assistant Resident General Surgery, 12 months |
| Year 5: Senior Resident Oral Surgery, 12 months |

degree track in 1971 and 1972 but were given individualized sequences because of the availability of positions in the medical school and general surgery program. One other resident, Michael Hauser, was accepted to the single-degree certificate program in 1978 with the intention of completing a dual-degree track. Dr. Guralnick helped him matriculate in medical school at University of Massachusetts because he did not attend HSDM and was not eligible for the Harvard MD program. Hauser did his general surgery training at the Deaconess Medical Center, a Harvard affiliated hospital.]

## Biography of Walter C. Guralnick

Walter Guralnick was born in East Boston on November 1, 1916 "in a home dedicated to issues of social justice and the principled delivery of universal health care" [6]. He attended Boston Latin School, where he met his future father-in-law, Philip Marson (one of his teachers), and through him his future wife, Betty. Upon graduation from Massachusetts State College (now University of Massachusetts), he went on to Harvard Dental School from which he graduated in 1941 [6].

At Harvard, he attended lectures by Dr. Varaztad H. Kazanjian "The Miracle Man of the Western Front" who achieved fame for his skill in treating the highly destructive and disfiguring facial injuries suffered by large numbers of British soldiers in World War I [7]. Following dental school, Guralnick chose to enroll in the Oral Surgery program at the Boston City Hospital (BCH) because it was a busy clinical service and it would also provide him with an excellent experience in anesthesia. He recalled doing anesthesia, at BCH, having expanded access because his brother, Eugene, was a Resident in General Surgery. While there, on the seventh December 1941, Pearl Harbor was attacked, and the US entered WWII. He remembered the moment: "… very vividly. I was up in the House Officer's Quarters in my room when, all of a sudden, the radio announced what had happened … I had anticipated that this was where we were going to go. There was no question that for many of us … but this was sort of our war" [8].

On January 1, 1942, he married Betty Marson. He completed his 1-year residency in June and then enlisted in the army as a dentist. He signed up with the 7th General Hospital although it had not yet been activated. He received orders, in July 1942, to report to Morris Air Force Base in Charlotte, North Carolina, where they had a dental clinic at the Base Hospital (Fig. 17.1). They were having problems with their OS program, so

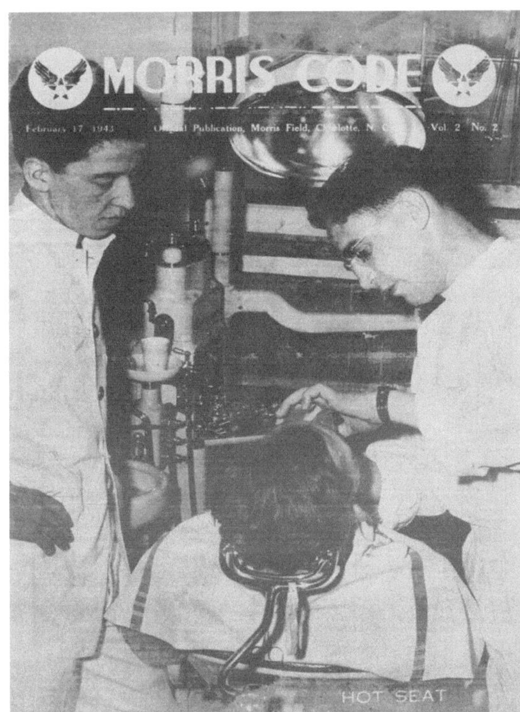


**Fig. 17.1** Dr. Guralnick, on patient's right, doing a procedure in the Dental Clinic at Morris Air Force Base, Charlotte, NC, prior to being shipped out to Europe. Cover: Morris Code, February 17, 1943, 2. (With permission Journal of the History of Dentistry)

he filled the void. "...it was really like an advanced residency. I had just tons of work to do. I had two rooms in which to operate and all the help I needed" [9].

Guralnick began scholarly writing early in his career and published his first papers in 1943 on Ludwig's Angina and on his experiences at an army post while in service [10, 11]. At the base, he learned from the orthopedic and ear, nose, and throat surgeons and was sent to the Walter Reed Hospital in Washington, District of Columbia (DC), in early 1943, for a course in maxillofacial surgery. He was in DC for approximately 6 months and during that time was promoted to Captain. When the 7th General Hospital was activated on June 10, 1943, he returned to Fort Devens, near Boston. From there, the unit was shipped out to the UK, arriving on December 15, 1943 [9], the day his son Peter was born [12].

Having docked in Liverpool, UK, the seventh General Hospital arrived at its wartime location in the village of Nocton, near Lincoln, in eastern England the following day. Its strength was 56 officers, 103 nurses, 1 warrant officer, and 505 enlisted men (Fig. 17.2). This site was located near the airfields in a largely flat area of the Fens (a coastal plain in eastern England). They set about "attacking the task of setting up a general hospital in a newly built, unfinished, and largely unequipped physical plant, under very trying conditions." During the Spring, concrete floored tents were constructed, increasing the total bed capacity to about 1200. The greatest difficulties were those of equipment and supply. Only a fraction of the essentials for running a hospital were available and a good portion of the resources were unfamiliar items. Basic equipment either had to be made or salvaged from the village dumps and some of the facilities had to be repurposed [9].

Not only were supplies lacking, but for weeks all attempts to get needed items delivered were fruitless; they were bogged down in the confusion and misunderstandings of the supply system. Despite these difficulties, the hospital was officially opened for patients on January 1, 1944. Since the army units in the vicinity were largely Air Force, about 75% of the patients were Air

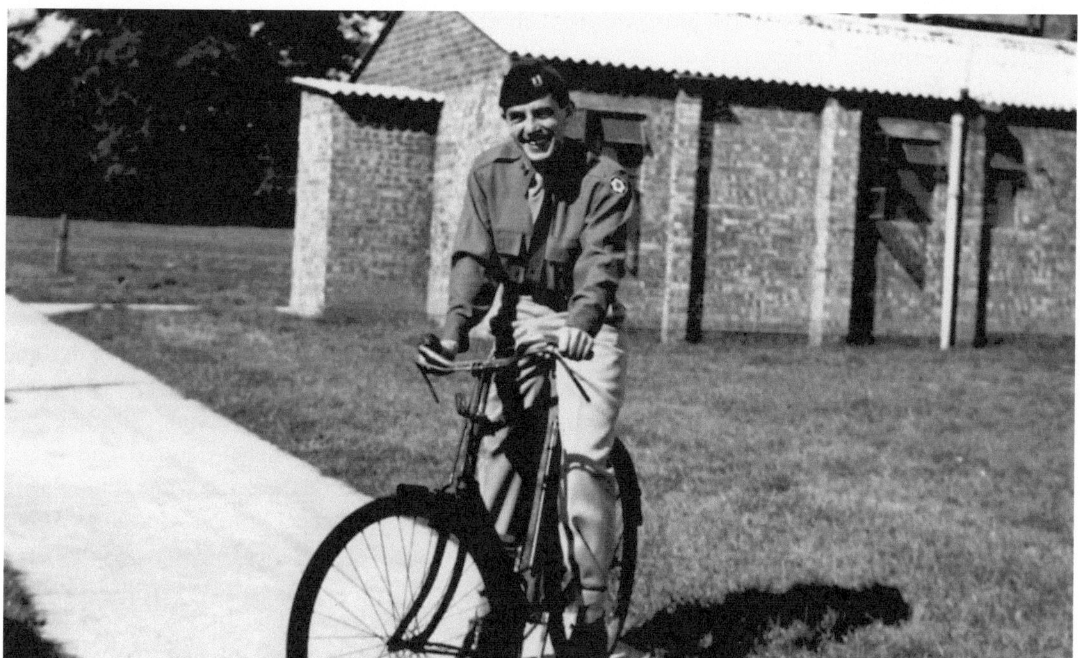

**Fig. 17.2** On his bicycle at seventh General Hospital, Nocton Air Force Base, Lincolnshire, UK (1944–1945). This appears to have been taken on a concrete path in front of the one-story brick wards. (Courtesy Tommy Guralnick. With permission Journal of the History of Dentistry)

Force personnel. In addition, several hundred battle casualties from Normandy (June 1944) were received by hospital trains and treated [9]. In his oral history, Guralnick was not very specific about the details of his work in the 7th Field Hospital. He recalled that they treated not only those who were injured but people who had other surgical problems such as cholecystitis, cholelithiasis, and appendicitis. However, he was also doing OS and some dentistry and developed an interest in skin grafting as most of the surgeons were not interested in this procedure [12] (Fig. 17.2).

In the latter part of the war, the army was faced with a critical shortage of satisfactory prosthetic eyes, needed for the wounded. The normal supply from Europe had been cut off and ordinary glass eyes had many disadvantages for military use: they were extremely fragile, were adversely affected by sudden changes in temperature and fluids in the eye socket, and required frequent replacement. Custom-fitted eyes required as many as 2 months for construction and some men lost up to 8 months duty in a single year while getting successive eye replacements. In addition, huge stocks of eyes were required for the proper fitting of a relatively smaller number of patients. As a result of this situation, several agencies undertook investigations to develop a prosthetic eye which would be readily available and superior to those made of glass. It is unclear as to who was the first to use methyl methacrylate [13], but the acrylic eye proved so superior that it was eventually adopted as the exclusive type of replacement by the army [14]. The part played by dental officers in creating these plastic eyes reflected great credit on the Dental Corps and the Medical Department. *The History of the 7th General Hospital* notes "The supplying of artificial eyes has been a considerable problem … and has been partially met by a technique employing plastics like those used in making certain dental appliances. Capt. Walter C. Guralnick, DC, of the Dental Service, has contributed to the development of this technique" [13]. Guralnick used his dental background and with available materials, known techniques and, no doubt, the talent of dental technicians to simply address this significant problem that confronted the wounded. The provision of well-fitting and esthetically pleasing prosthetic eyes would contribute greatly to the morale of the injured soldiers and their colleagues.

Modest to a fault, Guralnick rarely mentioned his contributions to the war effort, as was so often the case with men "just doing their jobs" under extraordinarily difficult conditions, far from home, loved ones, and support systems. He returned to Boston in 1946 and joined Dr. Harold Kent's successful oral surgery practice. Kent was a mentor to young Walter, but unfortunately, he died soon after Walter joined him. With some help from Mrs. Kent, Guralnick was able to purchase and successfully continue the practice. He joined the surgical staff at MGH in 1951 and the HSDM faculty in 1954. He was an active part-time faculty member, a favorite among students and was known for his surgical skills, interesting cases, and for his kind and empathetic manner as a surgeon, teacher, and mentor [6].

Upon the death of David Weissberger, then Chief of Oral Surgery and Dental Medicine at MGH, Guralnick was recruited and appointed Clinical Professor and Chief of the Oral Surgery Service at MGH (1967) and subsequently promoted to Professor of OMS in 1974. He served as Chief of OMS and Department Chair at HSDM from 1967 to 1982 and in 1987 was appointed Professor Emeritus. He was the first dentist to be awarded the Harvard Medal by President Lawrence Summers in 2005. The citation reads, in part: "Walter C. Guralnick, D.M.D. '41, has had an enormous influence on graduates of the Harvard School of Dental Medicine and the Harvard Medical School…. Through his demonstrated commitment to excellence, diversity and the ideals and goals of Harvard, the scope and place of dentistry in the teaching hospitals has dramatically changed. The Harvard and MGH community won't be the same without him" [6].

A first-class clinical scholar, Guralnick was a principal investigator on National Institutes of Health research and training grants, was awarded a Kellogg Foundation grant in 1996 to study delivery of health care, and authored numerous papers, book chapters, and books on a variety of subjects. Although a busy clinical surgeon, he always remained available and eager to help students, residents, and junior faculty. In recognition of his mentoring activities, he received the A. Clifford Barger Excellence in Mentoring Award from HMS in 2000. Guralnick served on the admissions committees of both HSDM and HMS and chaired the Committee on Promotions and Examinations at HSDM for 21 years [6].

At the MGH, Guralnick brought full recognition to OMS as a specialty by building a high volume, high-quality clinical service and a well-respected residency program. He is the only dentist to have chaired the General Executive Committee of the MGH. As the first Chairman of the Committee on Residency Education and Training of the AAOMS, he was instrumental in planning and implementing the OMFS In-service Training Examination (OMSITE). He was also a leader in attracting women and minorities into the profession. After 15 years as Chief of OMS, he stepped down and was appointed Director of the MGH Ambulatory Care Center and subsequently, Director of the Operating Rooms.

When asked what he considered his most important achievements, Guralnick replied modestly, first, changing the education of OMS for the better and second, helping to educate and train a cadre of superb leaders for our profession.

**Table 17.2** MGH, Harvard MD Oral and Maxillofacial Surgery Program: Started 1971, modified 1986, and in 1999 to 6 years for all residents [5, 15]

| | |
|---|---|
| Current form: | PGY 1, OMFS Intern 12 months |
| | PGY 2, Harvard Medical School third year |
| | PGY 3, Harvard Medical School fourth year |
| | (4 months anesthesia) |
| | PGY 4, MGH General Surgery Post Graduate Year (PGY) 2 level |
| | PGY 5, MGH General Surgery PGY 3 level |
| | (4 months, including 1 month Surgical Intensive Care Unit) |
| | OMFS Junior Resident 8 months |
| | PGY 6, OMFS Chief Resident, 4 months |
| | OMFS Senior Resident, 4 months |
| | Children's Hospital Senior, 4 months |

The first year and 20 months of the final 24 months remain an uninterrupted OMFS experience. Residents receive credit for 2 years general surgery

## Evolution of the Massachusetts General Hospital Harvard-MD Oral and Maxillofacial Surgery Program

The Harvard Program has evolved over the years as the Department, MGH and HMS gained more experience with the progress and outcomes of its trainees. From 1971 through 1985, the double-degree program was available, as written, only to Harvard dental students because they had the same curriculum as their medical school counterparts during the preclinical years [5, 15]. In 1986, acceptance of non-Harvard graduates was approved by HMS. These students were enrolled in a six-year program and had to complete the second year of the HMS curriculum (pathophysiology year) and the third year (principal clinical year). In 1999, based on changes in the HSDM and HMS curricula, all residents (Harvard and non-Harvard) were enrolled in a 6-year program beginning with the OS internship, then completing the third and fourth years of HMS prior to receiving the MD degree and returning to the residency program (Table 17.2). It is anticipated that there will be further changes in the coming years as the curricula in the medical and dental schools undergo significant changes. However, the department is committed to maintaining the 6-year template so as not to make the duration and cost of becoming an OMS prohibitive.

## Influence on OMFS Today

In 1971, there were two dual-degree OMS programs: MGH and University of Nebraska. By 2018 [16], 46/101 OMFS programs offered an MD track, i.e., dual degree and there were 1167 residents in training, 487 (42%) in an MD track [5]. The rise of double-degree programs and the increasing numbers of MD/general surgery trained OMSs have had a profound effect on the specialty. The scope of clinical practice has expanded with biomedical and bioengineering advances. In addition, the sophistication of OMFS training has increased with the advent of advanced specialty fellowships in head and neck oncology, pediatric/cleft and craniofacial surgery, temporomandibular joint surgery, minimally invasive surgery, and esthetic surgery. OMFS has gained increased recognition within hospitals, as well as the ACS. As mentioned above, both double-degree and single-degree surgeons have achieved fellowship in the ACS and now there is an OMFS section in the college. Recently, the fourth OMFS to be Chairman of the Joint Commission on Accreditation of Healthcare Organizations (JCAHO) has completed his term of office. The advances in OMFS education have in large part enabled these changes in status of the specialty. For this, we owe Guralnick a debt of gratitude for his vision and his courage to pursue it [5, 6].

## Discussion

### Challenges in the Future

Despite progress in OMS training, advent of dual-degree programs, advance training fellowships, increasing scope of practice, and increased recognition of the place of OMS as a legitimate surgical specialty by American dentistry, medicine, surgery, hospitals, insurance and government payors, and the primary American Surgery Organization (ACS), there are multiple challenges ahead.

Changes in medical education have resulted in new 4-year integrated, progressive programs including early exposure to patients, social sciences, health care economics, and delivery as well as the basic sciences and clinical patient care. This new concept of an integrated medical education has blurred the distinction that existed in traditional medical school curricula with years 1 and 2 devoted to basic science and years 3 and 4 to clinical patient care. The traditional curriculum provided a logical pathway for OMS residents who graduated from dental schools to transfer into medical schools for the third and fourth years to complete the required clinical training and receive the MD degree. In the current era, many medical schools no longer accept transfers into the third year and require that OMS residents enroll for 3 or even 4 years of medical school to obtain the MD degree. If this becomes the norm, there will be a tremendous financial burden on prospective OMS trainees with an additional 3–4 years of tuition over and above college and dental school. If our current residents graduate with $200,000 to $400,000 in debt, any increase may make OMS training untenable for many applicants.

Another potential challenge is the increasing number of states requiring 2 or 3 years of Accreditation Council for Graduate Medical Education (ACGME) training to qualify for a medical license. These challenges are in an environment where there is decreasing reimbursement for OMS services in hospitals and by insurance companies. This confluence of circumstances may completely disrupt the economics of OMS as a specialty and drive the debt (at the end of training) to income ratio (in the early years of practice) to an unacceptably high level [17]. Thus, it might become difficult to sustain the current system.

Solutions to the above challenges will have to be addressed in the long term and the outcomes are difficult to predict. However, the specialty of OMS would do well to follow the original principles of the Harvard Plan as described by Guralnick in the 1973 article [1]. The *duration* of residency training must be kept to a maximum total of 6 years to prevent loss of potential high-quality student applicants and residents who may choose other specialties. The pressure of new medical school curricula and difficulty of placing OMS residents as transfer students require that we find ways to integrate our trainees into medical school within a *total 6-year time frame, without compromising the OMS experience*. The problem of *increasing years of ACGME accredited post-MD training will need to be addressed*, perhaps by getting the ACGME to accredit OMS programs in collaboration with the Commission on Dental Accreditation. This may be possible now that the ACS accepts American Board of Oral and Maxillofacial Surgery certification as a benchmark credential for fellowship. Alternatively, working legislatively to get state medical boards to accept OMS training years for medical licensure, as they do for other specialties, otolaryngology, plastic surgery, orthopedics, neurosurgery, and urology, may be possible.

## Guralnick's Influence Beyond Massachusetts General and Harvard

Guralnick's influence went far beyond the confines of Boston and Harvard. In 1979, he established what became lasting relationships with colleagues in The People's Republic of China. In 1983, this broadened when a collaboration with Project Hope facilitated the exchange of Chinese doctors to the United States for expanded study. In addition, his leadership helped initiate the establishment of the first modern recovery rooms, comprehensive cleft/craniofacial teams, and state-of-the-art radiation therapy programs for head and neck cancer. These programs and personal relationships left an educational legacy and friendship between Chinese and American colleagues [6, 9] (Fig. 17.3).

In England, during World War II, he met Mr. Norman Rowe, a renowned British oral surgeon. Years later, with Rowe, Professor Geoffrey Howe, and Professor Malcolm Harris, he developed an exchange program between the MGH, Royal Dental/St. George's Hospitals, Roehampton, King's College, and the Eastman Dental Hospitals in England. British and American surgeons had their careers enhanced by this invaluable transatlantic rotation.

As Massachusetts Dental Society (MDS) President, Guralnick was instrumental in seeking legislative approval to establish the state's first public dental insurance program, the Massachusetts Dental Service Corporation which is now part of Delta Dental. He served as Chairman of the Massachusetts Board of Registration in Dentistry, President of the Massachusetts Society of Oral Surgeons, the MDS, and the New England Society of Oral Surgeons, in addition to founding the New England Foundation for Continuing Dental Education.

Guralnick's achievements have been recognized by numerous awards, including the previously mentioned Harvard Medal in 2005. He was a Senior Member of the Institute of Medicine of the National Academy of Sciences. He holds

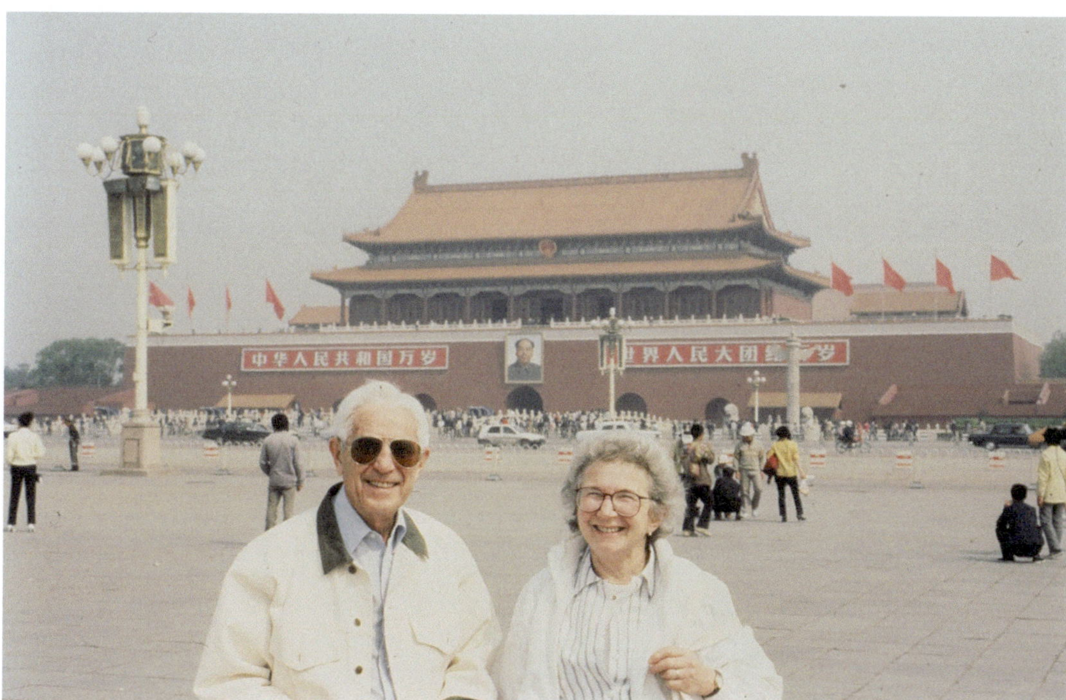


**Fig. 17.3** Walter and Betty Guralnick in front of the Forbidden City, Tiananmen Square, Beijing, China, circa early 1980s. (Courtesy Dr. Thomas Albert)

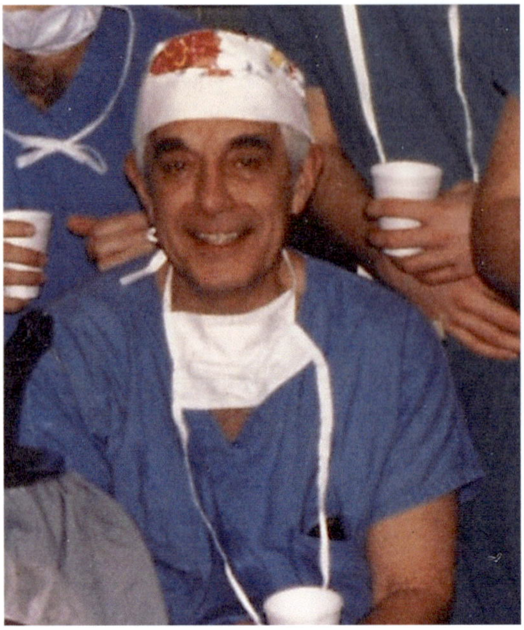

**Fig. 17.4** Guralnick after his last surgical case in the MGH Main Operating Rooms (1982). (Courtesy MGH Department of Oral and Maxillofacial Surgery)

honorary degrees from Xian Medical and West China Universities and was recognized by the Royal College of Surgeons of England with the award of an honorary fellowship for his contribution to international surgical training. The Walter C. Guralnick Professorship in OMS was established in 1993 at Harvard University and MGH. In 2009, Dr. Guralnick received the Arnold K. Maislen Award from the NYU College of Dentistry Department of Oral and Maxillofacial Surgery and the Gavel Medal from the Forsythe Institute in Boston for his contributions to OMS and dental research, respectively. He received numerous awards from the AAOMS during his career and the 96th Annual Meeting of the AAOMS (2014) was dedicated to Guralnick for his life-long contributions to the specialty (Figs. 17.4 and 17.5). Finally, his students are disproportionately represented in the ranks of senior and influential academic surgeons and leaders throughout the United States [5, 6, 15] (Figs. 17.6 and 17.7).

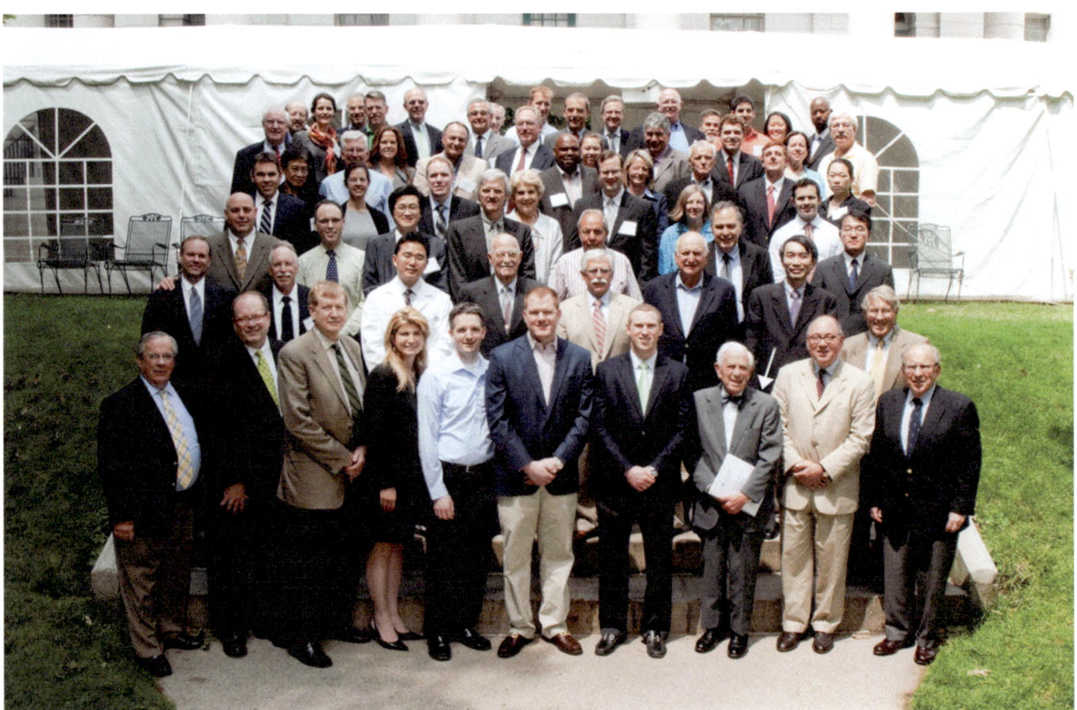

**Fig. 17.5** MGH Bicentennial Celebration OMS Symposium, June 2011. Department Photograph in front of Bullfinch Tent. Dr. Guralnick (in first row, arrow) with current residents, faculty, and alumni. (Courtesy MGH Photography Department)

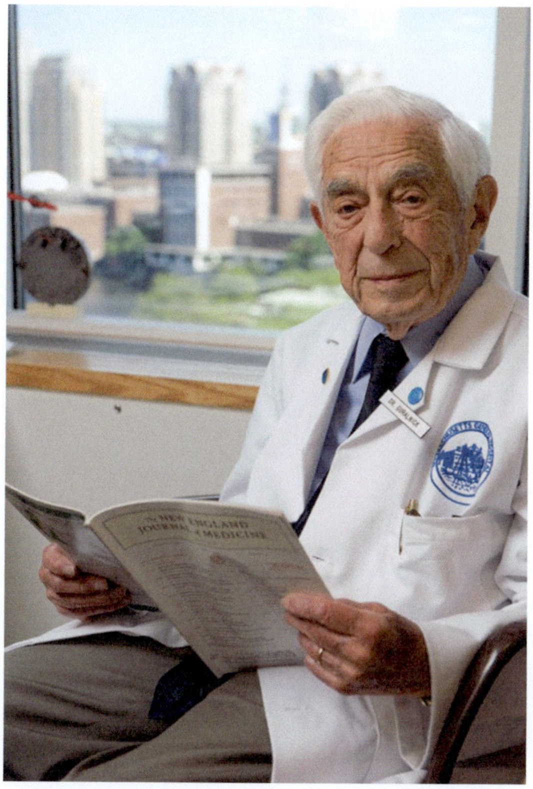

**Fig. 17.6** Dr. Guralnick, in his office in the MGH Warren Building circa 2013, reading his Journals as he often did during his trips to the hospital 2–3 times per week until his death, just short of his 101st birthday in 2017

Despite all his professional activities, Guralnick found the time to be a loving husband to Betty, his wife of 69 years, prior to her death in 2010, and a dedicated father to his 3 children (Peter, Susan, and Tommy). He had 5 grandchildren and, at the time of his death, 5 great-grandchildren. He took a personal interest in the lives and careers of his students and residents and was one of the most beloved faculty members of the Harvard School of Dental Medicine. "He is a wonderful human being, dedicated faculty member, and a true role model ... he provides thoughtful and caring one-to one clinical teaching and professional mentoring for students, residents, junior and even senior faculty" [18].

However, the words of his son Peter Guralnick an accomplished writer, biographer, and historian best describe the measure of the man that was Walter C. Guralnick. "All of the achievements for which he's been singled out today–all of those remarkable elements of a life that continues to be well lived, both personal and professional, are the very ones that Susan and Tommy and I have always recognized, from the time we were little kids. They are qualities of character most of all, qualities of principle and tenacity and public service, matters of dedication and conscience which were as much on display in the home as they were in his professional life." He goes on to describe his father's practice, "the orderliness was at the service of the patient. It was intended to set the patient at ease, and there was an unfailing sense of courtesy—*always*—an unwavering belief that the patient, not the doctor's dignity, was the focus." In summary, Peter concluded "I think this may have been the greatest lesson I took, and continue to take, from my father: There can be no distinction between your life and your work, assuming that your work is in fact your *profession* and not just a job. What remains so admirable to all of us in the family is that even at 99 the striving never stops. The striving for a better world, a better way to practice (and *deliver*) medicine. The ongoing commitment to a fairer, more just society. The abiding belief, certainly, not just in theory but in practice and in deed, that all of us are equal – but at the same time the recognition that those goals of fairness, of justice, of equality, will never be achieved unless we continue to commit ourselves to the struggle" [19]. It was these characteristics that made him so beloved, revered, and long remembered.

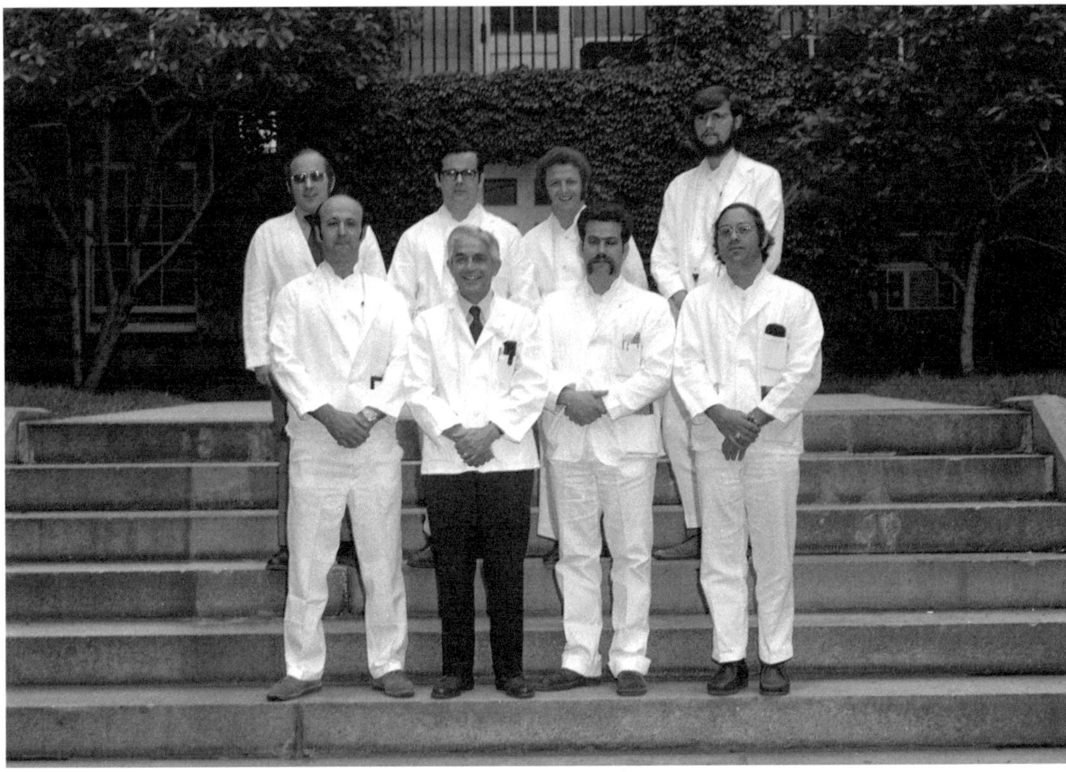

**Fig. 17.7** MGH Department of Oral and Maxillofacial Surgery 1971–1972 photograph. Bottom row (left-right): Robert Gracia (junior resident), Dr. Walter Guralnick, Edward Seldin, and Leonard Kaban (chief residents). Top row (left to right): RB Donoff (junior faculty), John PW Kelly (first enrolled intern), Hugh Ogus (rotating registrar from Roehampton, UK), Harry Schwartz (intern)

## References


1. Guralnick WC. The combined oral surgery-MD program: the Harvard plan. J Oral Surg. 1973;31(4):271–6. PMID: 4510650.
2. Alling CC, Hayward JR (co-editors): The building of a specialty: oral & maxillofacial surgery in the United States, 1918-1998. A supplement to the J Oral Maxillofac Surg. 1998. p. 120–121.
3. Hayward JR. The origin, extent and status of "Essentials of an adequate advanced training program in Oral Surgery". In: Proceedings of the fourth conference on graduate education in oral surgery. November 27, 1971, Chicago.
4. Shira RB. The specialty of oral surgery: present and future. J Oral Surg. 1969;27:286.
5. Kaban LB, Perrott DH. Dual-degree oral and maxillofacial surgery training in the United States: "Back to the future". J Oral Maxillofac Surg. 2020;78(1):18–28. https://doi.org/10.1016/j.joms.2019.08.026. Epub 2019 Sep 10. PMID: 31585062.
6. Kaban LB, Keith DA, Seldin EB, Albert TW. Dr Walter C. Guralnick Memorial Minute Harvard Medical School Annual Faculty Meeting Minutes, December 12th, 2018.
7. Deranian HM. Miracle man of the western front. Worcester, MA: Chandler House Press; 2007.
8. Walter Guralnick, DMD Oral History Video. Oral and Maxillofacial Surgery Chief Emeritus Massachusetts General Hospital 11/12/2007. Massachusetts General Hospital, Boston, MA. Accessed 8 Jan 2018.
9. Keith DA, Watson NAA, Kaban LB. Dr Guralnick's 'secret' mission. J Hist Dent. 2019;67(1):20–30. PMID: 32189636.
10. Williams AC, Guralnick WC. The diagnosis and treatment of Ludwig's Angina. N Engl J Med. 1943;28(14):444–50.
11. Guralnick WC. Experiences in exodontia and oral surgery at an army post. Am J Orthodont. 1943;29:241–6.
12. Guralnick P. My Father, … landed in England the day I was born and didn't return until I was more than two years old, nearly a year after V.E. Day. [5/8/45] http://www.peterguralnick.com/post/162860537671/reading-writing-real-life. Accessed 7 Dec 2018.

13. Role of the dental services in the development of the acrylic resin artificial eye. http://history.amedd.army.mil/corps/dental/wwii/chaptervi_wwii.html. p. 235. Last modified 12 Nov 2008.
14. Personal communication-email. Nolan A. (Andy) Watson 9/11/2018 AMEDD Center of History and Heritage, Fort Sam Houston, TX.
15. Dodson TB, Guralnick WC, Donoff RB, Kaban LB. Massachusetts General Hospital/Harvard Medical School MD Oral & Maxillofacial Surgery Program: a 30-year review. J Oral Maxillofac Surg. 2004;62:62–5.
16. American Association of Oral and Maxillofacial Surgeons Data, 2014–2018.
17. Asch DA, Nicholson S, Vujicic M. Are we in a medical education bubble market? N Engl J Med. 2013;369(21):1973–5. https://doi.org/10.1056/NEJMp1310778. Epub 2013 Oct 30. PMID: 24171508.
18. Personal Communication. Biographical sketch 2008. Courtesy Peter Guralnick.
19. Guralnick, P. 'About Walter Guralnick' HSDM honors 2016. Courtesy Peter Guralnick.

# 18 Orthognathic Surgery and a Tale of How Three Procedures Came to Be: A Letter to the Next Generation of Surgeons. Clinics of Plastic Surgery. Volume 34, Pages 331–355, 2007

Timothy A. Turvey

**Abstract**

Professor Hugo Obwegeser is considered the father of modern maxillofacial surgery. He created and perfected the sagittal split osteotomy and genioplasty, designed instrumentation still used today, and trained countless surgeons worldwide. What he left at the end of his career, published 10 years prior to his passing, was a memoir of how modern orthognathic surgery was developed.

**Keywords**

Orthognathic surgery · Sagittal split osteotomy · Genioplasty · Maxillofacial surgery

What would motivate a retired surgeon, in the twilight of his life to craft an article like this in a non-native language? Was it to relive the glory days or to remind the future generation of craniomaxillofacial surgeons that they have a responsibility to continue the legacy that they have inherited? A casual glance of the article suggests the former. A careful read, however, uncovers the motivation to be the latter. The last two sentences of the article make it clear that Obwegeser is sending a message and a reminder "Few procedures can alter the human face so fundamentally as these three procedures. I hope that these words will continue to inspire the generation of surgeons to follow." Interwoven throughout the article are subtle and poignant messages, some surgical, some professional, and some social.

Hugo Obwegeser, the most celebrated craniomaxillofacial surgeon of his time, left a legacy of being able to identify reconstructive surgical problems of the face and jaws and innovating, developing, and popularizing techniques to address the problems (Fig. 18.1). He will be remembered for his ability to methodically diagnosis, innovate and plan surgery, his surgical skills, his caring for patients, and educating others and the next generation of craniomaxillofacial surgeons. Very importantly, he shared his thoughts, views, and experiences by lecturing, publishing, and making friends worldwide. Obwegeser was the founder of the European Association of Craniomaxillofacial Surgeons and the first editor of the journal. He was a leader and was able to unite a fragmented group of surgeons of similar interests but of different cultures, ethnicity, race, and languages.

T. A. Turvey (✉)
Department of Oral and Maxillofacial Surgery, University of North Carolina, Chapel Hill, NC, USA
e-mail: Tim_Turvey@unc.edu



S. R. Aziz, M. D. Turner (eds.), *Classic Papers and Pioneers in Maxillofacial and Oral Surgery*,
https://doi.org/10.1007/978-3-031-63246-4_18

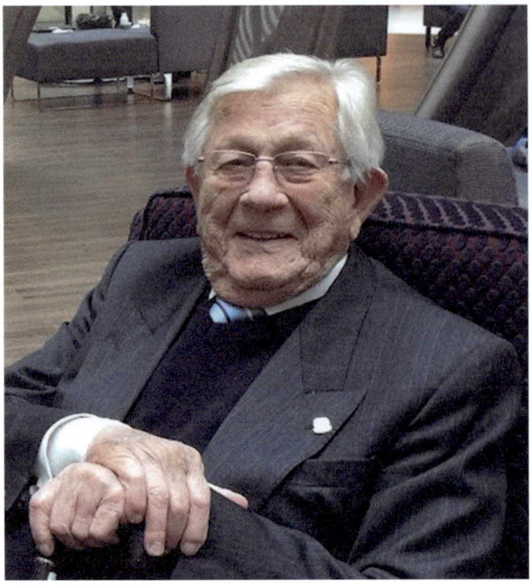

**Fig. 18.1** Professor Obwegeser circa 2015

English was not his primary language nor was it the primary language of many Europeans, but he recognized that communication was important for the advancement of the surgical specialty and was able to convince others of this. He mastered the language and insisted that all presentations at the European Association of Craniomaxillofacial Surgeons' meetings and all papers published in the *Journal of Craniomaxillofacial Surgery* be in English.

A survivor of World War II and living in post-war Austria were challenges, but they provided Obwegeser opportunities to learn from very experienced surgeons who were advanced in their careers, especially with reconstructing trauma and war casualties. He often credited his mentors and his contemporaries for stimulating and influencing him. Similarly, he acknowledged some of his trainees including Emil Steinhauser and Herman Sailer and makes references to other surgeons who described modifications of his techniques (Hunsuck, Bell, Epker, etc.). He embraced technology and its influence on maxillofacial surgery, but he adopted it strategically and always after it had proven itself. Early in his career, he recognized the limitations of surgery of the face with anesthesia, lighting, surgical access, and inadequate instrumentation. Unwilling to accept these limitations, Obwegeser challenged the developers of anesthetic techniques, worked with instrument manufacturers to develop appropriate equipment, and used his imagination and ingenuity to improve the conditions for performing these procedures.

Sagittal osteotomy of the mandible, genioplasty via pedicled horizontal osteotomy of the symphysis, and LeFort I osteotomy are the workhorses of orthognathic surgery. In this manuscript, Obwegeser chronicles his involvement in the development and application of these procedures. Methodically, Obwegeser was able to identify a clinical problem and develop a plan for resolving it. He possessed the ability to assimilate experiences and utilized his background, training, previous surgical exposures, and creativity to solve surgical challenges of the face and jaws. Throughout the manuscript, Obwegeser stresses the importance of imagination and creativity.

The manuscript provides an insight into Obwegeser's methodical approach to problem identification and solving and his innovativeness and creativity with developing surgical techniques. He explains how he used his experience in treating fractures to help bridge the links with developing orthognathic surgical techniques including the sagittal osteotomy, the muscular pedicled genioplasty, and the LeFort I osteotomy via the intraoral approach. He was an advocate of using transoral incisions and minimizing facial scars to approach maxillofacial surgical problems. Later in his career, he adopted the coronal approach when conducting upper face osteotomies. Obwegeser credits his mentor, Professor Richard Trauner, the former chairman of maxillofacial surgery at the University of Gratz for instilling in him the fervor for maxillofacial surgery and addressing the many challenges of this patient population. After beginning his career as an unpaid assistant to Professor Arnold Chiarri, a Viennese pathologist, Obwegeser developed appreciation for knowing and understanding pathophysiology. Chiarri also taught him to think and to explore. By 1947, Obwegeser was invited to become a paid assistant by Trauner in Gratz, where he trained and where he remained until

1958. Trauner and Obwegeser coauthored many manuscripts. In 1958, he joined the faculty at the University of Zurich School of Medicine and became Head of the Department of Maxillofacial Surgery where he spent his career until 1987. During his years with Trauner, Obwegeser was able to visit multiple other maxillofacial surgery units where he learned different surgical techniques including soft tissue surgery. The time spent with Sir Harold Gilles in London, Eduard Schmidt in Stuttgart, and Hans Pichler in Vienna were invaluable experiences that shaped his career. These rotations also allowed him to develop collegial and lifetime relationships with contemporaries such as Norman Rowe, Karl Hogeman, Ivo Pitanguay, Ralph Millard, and Paul Tessier. He built the Department of Maxillofacial Surgery in Zurich to become a world-famous center of excellence for maxillofacial surgery.

Recanting his initial experiences with sagittal osteotomies and the difficulties encountered during the procedure, the on-the-spot decision making to alter the surgical plan and the patient's postoperative course, teaches us about Obwegeser, the person. Complications did not deter him. He believed in himself enough to see his way through a plan that many others would have abandoned. He persisted, persevered, and managed. Importantly, he learned from his experiences and altered techniques and osteotomy designs over time. He was open to others' insights and willingness to try them as long as they made sense. Obwegeser credited others, such as Perthes and Schlossman, whose works inspired his thoughts on the development of sagittal osteotomy and Dal Pont, Bell, and Epker for suggesting modifications that made sense to him. He gave credit, where credit was due. In this article, Obwegesser acknowledges the contributions of Hans Luhr with the development of bone plates and screws, which he adopted later in his career.

Obwegeser describes the evolution of the sagittal osteotomy from its infancy (confined to the vertical ramus) to its latter design (through the body of the mandible). He emphasizes (by citing exceptions) the importance of pre-planning and that not all patients are the same. Modifications must be made to accommodate to the patient's anatomy and conditions. He describes a particular patient with a long, slender mandible and a neurovascular bundle that was at high risk of severing with the conventional sagittal osteotomy operation. Cleverly, he designed the patient's procedure to include the removal of the buccal cortex of the mandible from the vertical ramus to the body, repositioning the neurovascular bundle, an angle osteotomy through the remaining lingual cortex, repositioning the segments, and then replacing and securing the buccal cortex to stabilize the complex. He combined this procedure with a posterior maxillary osteotomy to close an open bite. This was not treatment planning in the operating room, but careful and methodical planning done prior to surgery. Although not stated in this article, for many years Obwegeser shunned posterior maxillary osteotomy, citing Schuchardt's experience with relapse. The acknowledgement of the use of the posterior maxillary osteotomy to close an open bite demonstrates his acceptance of the works of other credible surgeons who had favorable results with the procedure and his eventual acceptance of the procedure.

Obwegeser was beyond carpentry. He understood the interaction of muscle activity on bone as is demonstrated by the sagittal osteotomy design to reduce the stresses placed on the muscles of mastication, especially the temporalis. He understood bone healing and he recognized the importance of having a broad surface of cancellous bone contact to improve healing. He stresses the importance of a period of immobilization and fixation of the segments. He recognized the importance of occlusion and mentions equilibration of teeth to assist in achieving a favorable outcome. Unfortunately, he did not have access to orthodontists until the latter part of his career and therefore occlusal equilibration was something that he performed himself. Throughout the article, Obwegeser stresses the importance of good bone contact with osteotomy design, transoral incisions without facial scarring, and securing the segments in place with suture or wire. He relied on intermaxillary fixation for stabilization of osteotomies until he finally adopted bone plates and screws which came along later in his career.

A clear message to the next generation of maxillofacial surgeons included in this article is to acknowledge credit to others for their pioneering experiences and not to plagiarize the works of others or ignore others' contributions to the same topic. Obwegeser acknowledged Dal Ponts' modification of the sagittal osteotomy but speaks poignantly of the publication of the modification without acknowledgement of him and knowing that Dal Pont never performed the procedure. He also cites Schuchardt for performing and publishing on sagittal osteotomy without crediting him. Apparently Schuchardt was present in Gratz when Obwegeser performed his second sagittal osteotomy in 1954. Schuchardt returned to Hamburg and performed the procedure, published it, but never gave credit to Obwegeser. Obwegeser was a stickler for historical details in publications and presentations.

Obwegesser knew well and understood the problems of altering the projection of the chin with free bone grafts and allografts. He recognized the limitations of free bone grafts (resorption) to alter the chin and with the use of alloplast (infection, bone and dental root resorption, displacement, etc.). Utilizing a technique that was published by a pre-war predecessor, Hofer, who Obwegeser suspected performed the procedure on a cadaver only, Obwegeser developed the procedure during a presurgical planning session with cephalometric tracings and published the results in 1957. Using his extensive previous experience with trauma victims, he designed the intraoral approach to alter the chin via a vestibular and lip incision and avoided skin incisions. Emphasizing the importance of the mental nerve and its preservation and maintaining soft tissue and muscular attachments to the mobilized segment as well as stabilization of the segment with a dental splint initially and suture material later, he stresses basic surgical principles.

Obwegeser addressed the issues of midface surgery by designing instrumentation to assist in sectioning the maxilla, developing instrumentation to assist with mobilization, and developed techniques to assist with stabilization, using bone grafts, sutures, wires, etc. With LeFort I osteotomy, Obwegeser recants his experience of observing Gilles and Rowe perform lateral mobilization of the cleft maxilla through vestibular incisions. He recalls that Gilles never advanced a cleft maxilla but relied on mandibular setback to achieve appropriate occlusion. He credits the works of Wassmund and Auxhausen who published extensively on osteotomy designs and complete mobilization of the entire maxilla and advancement for a variety of conditions. He makes references to the early works of von Langenbeck and Cheever who used facial incisions for tumor access to the maxilla and nasopharynx via maxillary osteotomies. Although others may have performed LeFort I osteotomies before him, it was Obwegeser who modified, inspired, and promoted the acceptance of these operations. His published works stimulated many surgeons worldwide to begin offering these procedures to the patients for whom they were responsible. His early works inspired people like William Bell to investigate the revascularization and wound healing of the maxilla following LeFort I osteotomy with perfusion studies on primates. He emphasizes the importance of complete mobilization of the maxilla, releasing scar tissue, and using free bone grafts in the osteotomy defects. His initial experience was with cleft patients and post-trauma patients; however, Obwegeser quickly applied these techniques to developmental and congenital malformations as well.

Recognizing the limitations of mandibular surgery alone (esthetic) and ignoring the problem of maxillary deficiency in many patients lead Obwegeser to develop the maxillary osteotomy, especially involving those of retromaxillism. This occurred in the 1960s and by the 1970s Obwegeser recognized the importance of simultaneous mobilization of both jaws. Although he describes using his intraoperative judgment to assist in knowing where to reposition the jaws, he later described the importance of presurgical planning with articulated study models, cephalometric tracings, and constructed splints to assist with the intraoperative positioning of the jaws.

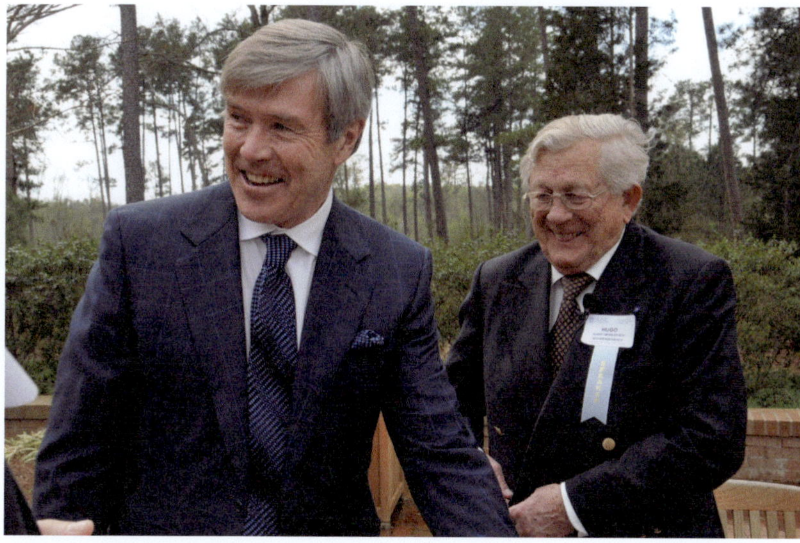

**Fig. 18.2** Dr. Timothy Turvey and Professor Obwegeser

Obwegeser's message in this article is clear. With difficulty lies opportunity. Education, background, training, and experience are essential to allow us to do what we do today. It is ability to recognize a problem, creativity, and ingenuity that will allow us to take craniomaxillofacial surgery to the next level (Fig. 18.2).

# Le Forte 1 Osteotomy for Correction of Maxillary Deformities. Journal of Oral Surgery. Vol 33, June 1975

19

Eric Reimer and Shahid R. Aziz

**Abstract**

Within the wide scope of oral and maxillofacial surgery, orthognathic surgery is considered one of the cornerstone specialties an oral and maxillofacial surgery can provide for patient care. Not only does orthognathic surgery provide esthetic benefits for patients but more importantly improving function by correcting the dentofacial deformity. The first large technical advancements in this area of surgery came in the twentieth century in Europe. However, Dr. William Bell was an American oral and maxillofacial surgeon pioneering the study of wound healing, vascularity, and surgical biology of maxillary and mandibular osteotomies. Notably, he provided over 170 journal articles, 8 textbooks, and countless book chapters to further the study of orthognathic surgery and correction of dentofacial deformities. One of his early papers in the year 1975 describing the vascularity, wound healing, and technique for the modern maxillary Le Forte or Le Fort I osteotomy still holds true and continues to be practiced today.

**Keywords**

Maxillary osteotomy · Le Fort osteotomy · Orthognathic surgery · Dentofacial deformity · Maxillofacial surgery

E. Reimer
Oral and Maxillofacial Surgery, Hackensack Meridian Health, Edison, NJ, USA

S. R. Aziz (✉)
Division of Oral and Maxillofacial Surgery, Department of Otolaryngology, Hackensack Meridian School of Medicine, Nutley, NJ, USA
e-mail: azizsr@sdm.rutgers.edu; Shahid.aziz@hmhn.org

The Le Fort(e) I osteotomy or previously referred to as the "total maxillary osteotomy" remains the primary workhorse osteotomy for correction of maxillary dentofacial deformities in current practice today. This technique utilizes osteotomes to separate the maxilla along certain junctions to allow complete mobilization and repositioning of the maxilla into a new position to correct these facial and occlusal disharmonies. It developed its name from the classic studies by French surgeon René Le Fort in 1901, who observed the midface fracture patterns following blunt trauma. Le Fort used a variety of objects such as clubs, pipes, cannon balls to recreate the blunt facial trauma seen in military field hospitals. From his studies, he concluded three common fracture schemes which were Le Fort I, II, and III respective of the involvement of the maxilla and naso-orbitoethmoid complex. Le Fort also noted that a pterygoid fracture is highly specific in these fracture patterns (Fig. 19.1). The modern Le Fort I



S. R. Aziz, M. D. Turner (eds.), *Classic Papers and Pioneers in Maxillofacial and Oral Surgery*,
https://doi.org/10.1007/978-3-031-63246-4_19

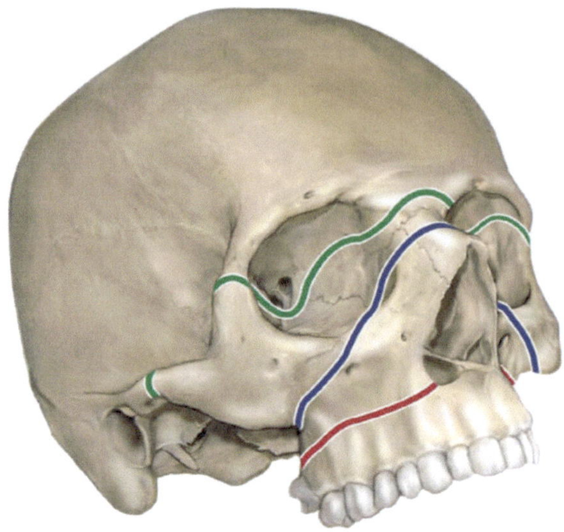


**Fig. 19.1** Le Fort type and classification of fracture patterns

elective osteotomy used for correction of midface deficiencies recreates a true Le Fort I fracture pattern for maxillary mobilization and establishment of new facial and occlusal harmony and is so such named.

The modernization of the current practice of the Le Fort I osteotomy was a result of many surgeons across different surgical specialties. The horizontal osteotomy apical to the maxillary teeth was first described by German surgeon Bernhard von-Langenbeck in 1859 to access nasopharyngeal pathology. Several years later in 1867, David Cheever performed a similar operation to access nasopharyngeal pathology but did so bilaterally in the maxilla and was termed the "double operation." It was not until 1927 when Martin Wassmund performed the modern day Le Fort I osteotomy for correction of an anterior open bite. However, he did not fully mobilize the maxilla but instead used orthopedic traction with elastics to close the occlusion. From this point until the beginning of the 1950s, multiple surgeons attempted the Le Fort I osteotomy with trial-and-error modifications. It was noted that the area of the pterygoid plates was difficult to osteotomize without fully mobilizing the maxilla and also came with a high risk of encountering bleeding. For example, Schuchardt in 1942 attempted a staged approach where he performed a horizontal maxillary osteotomy apical to the teeth and placed the patient in traction with overhead weights. Then several weeks later, he performed osteotomies of the pterygoid plates as to have time for revascularization of the maxilla from his initial osteotomy.

The common theme during this time was that maxillofacial surgeons were not able to fully move the maxilla to the desired amount and relapse was common. As maxillofacial surgeons did not fully understand the perfusion and vascular supply to the maxilla and did not want the maxilla to necrose intraoperatively or in the postoperative period. It was Obwegeser who recognized this in the late 1950s and began implementing more aggressive advancements of the maxilla following the Le Fort I osteotomy. He (Obwegeser) had noticed that, Gillies and Rowe, in multiple cleft cases for maxillary surgery, would create green-stick fractures at the pterygomaxillary junction and rotate the cleft segments inferiorly. Then the mandible was set back with osteotomies to correct the occlusion, and Obwegeser noted that the patients retained their "dish face" and "flat appearance" as the maxilla was still deficient.

As Obwegeser continued his surgical innovation of the total maxillary osteotomy, he began to treat a higher number of cleft patients and posttraumatic facial deformities with greater degrees of maxillary advancement. In 1968, he advanced the maxilla of a cleft patient 13 mm and noted the complete fracture and mobilization of the segments was key to establishing the occlusion. He also realized with these large advancements that the blood supply of the maxilla was robust and resilient to large horizontal circumvestibular incisions and complete separation of the maxilla from the cranial base. It was in 1969 that Obwegeser completed the first simultaneous bilateral sagittal split osteotomies of the mandible in conjunction with the Le Fort I total maxillary osteotomy that was fixated with interosseous wiring, bone grafts, and intermaxillary fixation for 6 weeks. He utilized cephalometric tracings and radiographs to develop a treatment plan that would allow him to establish the correct occlusion while also correcting facial disharmonies. Several small alterations to the Le Fort I osteotomy have occurred since this initial "orthognathic" procedure, and in addition to the advent of internal fixation with plates and screws in the 1970s, the modern Le Fort 1 osteotomy was born.

After Obwegeser modernized and demonstrated the success of the Le Fort I osteotomy, there were several maxillofacial surgeons who investigated the biological foundation of orthognathic surgery. The most prominent in this research was William H. Bell (Fig. 19.2). Starting in the 1970s, he provided the foundational studies and answers many of the surgeons at the time were asking, such as wound and bone healing of the maxilla, vascular stability, and revascularization following osteotomies. Bell began developing a microangiographic and histologic technique first with rabbits in pilot studies, which later progressed to larger mammal studies utilizing rhesus monkeys, dogs, and baboons to better understand jaw osteotomies. Overall, there were a total of 9 major animal studies from 1969 to 1995 in which Bell evaluated all the maxillary and mandibular osteotomies used in modern orthognathic surgery to validate their wound healing and revascularization.

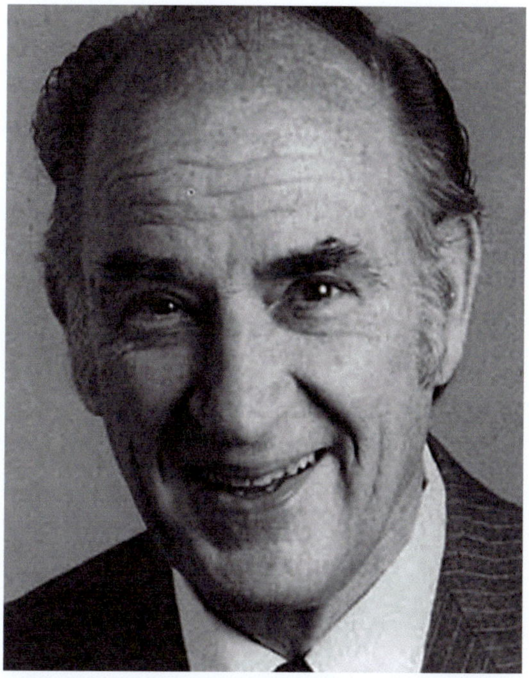

**Fig. 19.2** Dr. William H Bell (March 28, 1927–June 1, 2016)

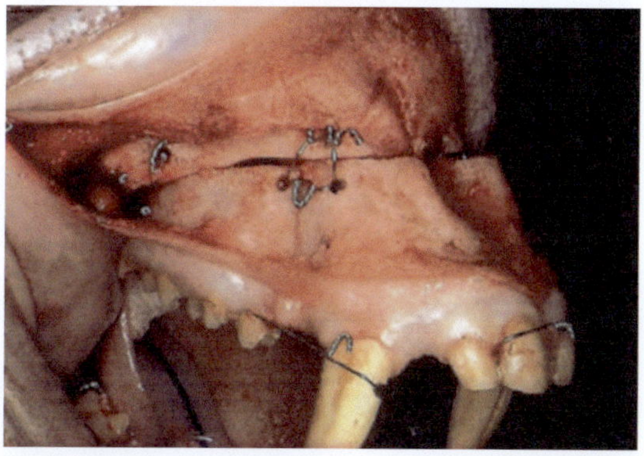

**Fig. 19.3** Rhesus monkey subject with replicated maxillary Le Fort I osteotomy with down-fracture and mobilization and internal wire fixation

Bell's most notable vascular and wound healing study was published in 1975 looking at Le Fort I or total maxillary osteotomy; the same year he published his revolutionary clinical case series article that is the focus of this chapter. His total maxillary osteotomy wound healing study utilized rhesus monkeys in which a Le Fort I osteotomy was performed via a circumvestibular incision and mobilized as Obwegeser previously described and fixated with trans osseous wires (Fig. 19.3). In a subset of the experimental group, the descending palatine arteries were ligated and transected. The experimental and control groups were then sacrificed at different time intervals to include immediately after surgery, 2 days, 1, 2, 4, 6, and 12 weeks after the operation. Following sacrifice, the carotid arteries of the animals were exposed, heparinized, and then injected with radiopaque dye. This allowed Bell to evaluate the osteotomized maxilla via histologic and microangiographic techniques (Fig. 19.4).

This study concluded that there was not a sole blood vessel that was responsible for perfusing the maxilla, and that collateral circulation of the ascending palatine and ascending pharyngeal provided a robust blood supply, thus, allowing the maxilla to be down-fractured and mobilized using a circumvestibular incision. Furthermore, ligation and transection of the descending palatine arteries was of little significance and only caused short-term and temporary disturbance of perfusion to the maxillary pulpal, osseous, and soft tissues. It was also observed in this study that at as early as 4 weeks following the operation there was callus formation and by 6 weeks areas of mature bone configuration along the osteotomy segments. Bell continued to build from this work and show that the maxilla could also be segmented in the anterior and posterior regions following a Le Fort I down-fracture with similar vascular and wound healing results in an animal model. These experimental studies provided the biological foundation for maxillofacial surgeons that instilled confidence to continue to develop these techniques for correction of traumatic and congenital dentofacial deformities.

In addition to Bell's laboratory research, he also developed clinical studies and produced a landmark article in 1975 describing the clinical applications and techniques of the Le Fort I osteotomy. The article titled "The Le Forte I Osteotomy for Correction of Maxillary Deformities" is a cornerstone paper in the oral and maxillofacial literature in which Bell provided technical notes of the operation and atlas photographs/figures modernizing Obwegeser total maxillary osteotomy technique. The article presents a series of 15 patients with either cleft, post-traumatic, or congenital skeletofacial deformities treated by Bell from 1971 to 1975 with this specific operation (Table 19.1). Bell begins the article by describing the history of the operation and touches on his translational research that provided the biological groundwork for this maxillary operation, which is mentioned previously in this chapter.

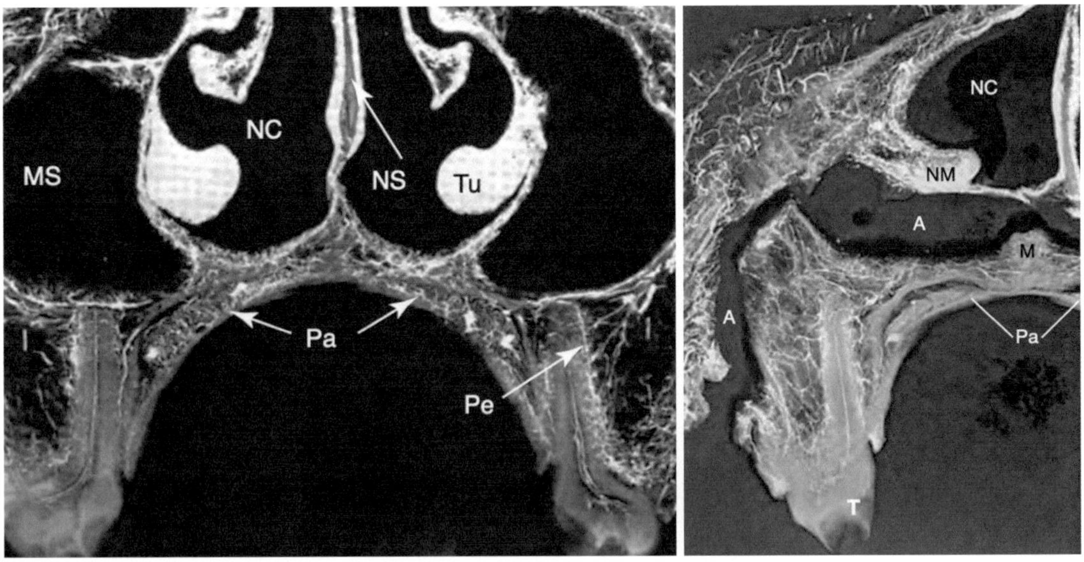


**Fig. 19.4** Microangiographic studies. Coronal sections of microangiogram study of the maxilla from control animal (left) versus total maxillary osteotomy subject (right) taken from Bell's study. *A* avascular space, *M* maxilla, *MS* maxillary sinus, *NC* nasal cavity, *NS* nasal septum, *Pa* palate, *Pe* periodontal vascular plexus, *T* tooth, *Tu* inferior turbinate

**Table 19.1** Treatments used to correct deformities of the maxilla in 15 patients since 1971

| Case no. | Age | Race | Sex | Dental facial deformity[a] | Etiology | Movement of maxilla (mm) | Treatment[b] | Complications | Follow-up (months) |
|---|---|---|---|---|---|---|---|---|---|
| 1 | 16 | W | M | MR | Developmental | Anterior, 10 | 1, 2, 4 | None | 29 |
| 2 | 21 | W | F | MAH | Developmental | Superior, 7 | 1 | None | 3 |
| 3 | 21 | W | F | MR, MP | Developmental | Anterior, 6 | 1, 2, 4, 6, 7 | Posterior open bite | 29 |
| 4 | 19 | W | M | MR, AOB | Cleft lip and palate | Anterior, 9 | 1, 2, 3, 4 | Widening of alar base | 29 |
| 5 | 44 | W | M | MR | Posttraumatic | Anterior, 10 | 1, 5 | None | 32 |
| 6 | 32 | B | F | MR | Posttraumatic | Anterior, 9 | 1, 2 | None | 16 |
| 7 | 20 | W | F | MAH | Developmental | Posterior, 4<br>Superior, 6 | 1 | Flattening of upper lip | 5 |
| 8 | 16 | W | M | MR | Cleft lip and palate | Anterior, 12<br>Lateral, 6 | 1 | Relapse | 15 |
| 9 | 19 | B | F | BP, MAH, AOB | Developmental | Superior, 10 | 1, 6 | None | 6 |
| 10 | 18 | W | M | MR | Cleft lip and palate | Anterior, 13 | 1, 2 | None | 8 |
| 11 | 26 | W | F | MAH | Developmental | Posterior, 15<br>Superior, 5 | 1 | None | 13 |
| 12 | 25 | W | F | MAH, AOB | Developmental | Superior, 7<br>Posterior, 4 | 1, 3, 4 | None | 13 |
| 13 | 23 | W | F | AOB | Idiopathic | Superior, 10 | 1, 3, 7 | Widening of alar base | 5 |
| 14 | 20 | W | M | MR | Posttraumatic | Anterior, 4 | 1, 3, 5, 7 | None | 12 |
| 15 | 17 | W | F | MAH, AOB | Developmental | Superior, 6 | 1, 3, 4 | None | 14 |

[a] Key: *AOB* anterior open bite, *MAH* maxillary alveolar hyperplasia, *BP* bimaxillary protrusion, *MR* maxillary retrusion, *MP* mandibular prognathism
[b] Key: (1) Total maxillary osteotomy, (2) Bone graft, (3) Genioplasty, (4) Orthodontics, (5) Malar contouring, (6) Mandibular osteotomy, (7) Rhinoplasty

Next, Bell describes the anesthesia required for the operation as well as an in-depth protocol for the surgical technique. He mentions the use of hypotensive anesthesia during maxillary surgery to aid in the reduction of submucosal oozing and states that the "technical skill and experience of the anesthesiologist must be of a high order." He then proceeds to describe the access to the maxilla and the various osteotomies to separate the maxilla from the cranial base for mobilization. These osteotomies include the horizontal supra-apical, lateral nasal wall, nasal septum, and pterygoid plates (Fig. 19.5). Once the maxilla is mobilized after the osteotomies, he notes in the technical notes that the maxilla should be so mobile that only light finger pressure can move the maxilla to the desired position. The maxilla is then placed into the desired occlusion based on the previously made index/splint and the patient is placed into maxillomandibular fixation for 6–8 weeks. Plate fixation was not prevalent during this time and Bell recommended using trans-osseous wire fixation between the osteotomy sites or infra-orbital rim and circumzygomatic suspension wires, when possible, to further fixate the maxilla in the new position. Furthermore, he comments that bone grafting is not routinely required for adequate osseous healing but can be considered in large transverse or advancement movements and in cleft patients. During this technical section, he also describes the numerous modifications for

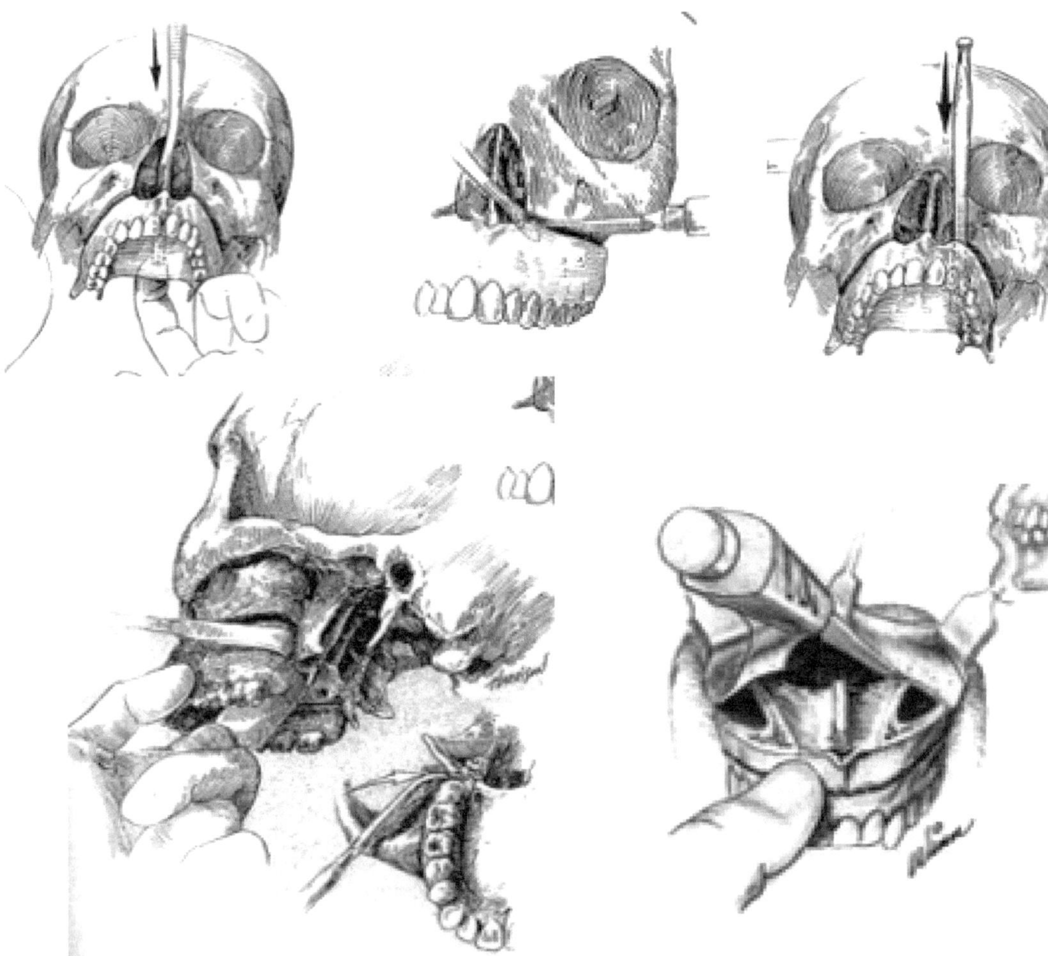

**Fig. 19.5** Renderings from Bell's publication illustrating the osteotomy sites for complete maxillary osteotomy or Le Fort I osteotomy

maxillary impactions and correcting transverse relationships with segmentation of the maxilla (Fig. 19.6).

The next section of the article describes the applications of this technique. Specifically, Bell describes cases of maxillary hypoplasia, cleft deformities, apertognathia, post-traumatic facial deformities that were treated to correct the facial skeleton and malocclusion (Table 19.1). In addition to treatment with the Le Fort I osteotomy, he also notes that adjunctive procedures or therapies were utilized in creating ideal treatment outcomes for his patients. These included malar augmentation, pre-surgical and post-surgical orthodontics, rhinoplasty, genioplasty, bone grafting. Figure 19.7 gives a case example from Bell's article showing the preoperative and postoperative clinical photos and cephalometric tracings exhibiting excellent esthetic results and correction of the skeletofacial deformity and malocclusion.

Throughout this section of his case presentations in the article, Bell also divulges several clinical pearls from his work. Many of which have become staples in modern orthognathic textbooks and still taught today to residents in training. These clinical concepts are listed below as direct quotes or as paraphrases.

- "An obtuse nasolabial angle is probably the single most important diagnostic criterion for total maxillary advancement. The upper lip-nose balance can be significantly improved by reduction of such an angle."

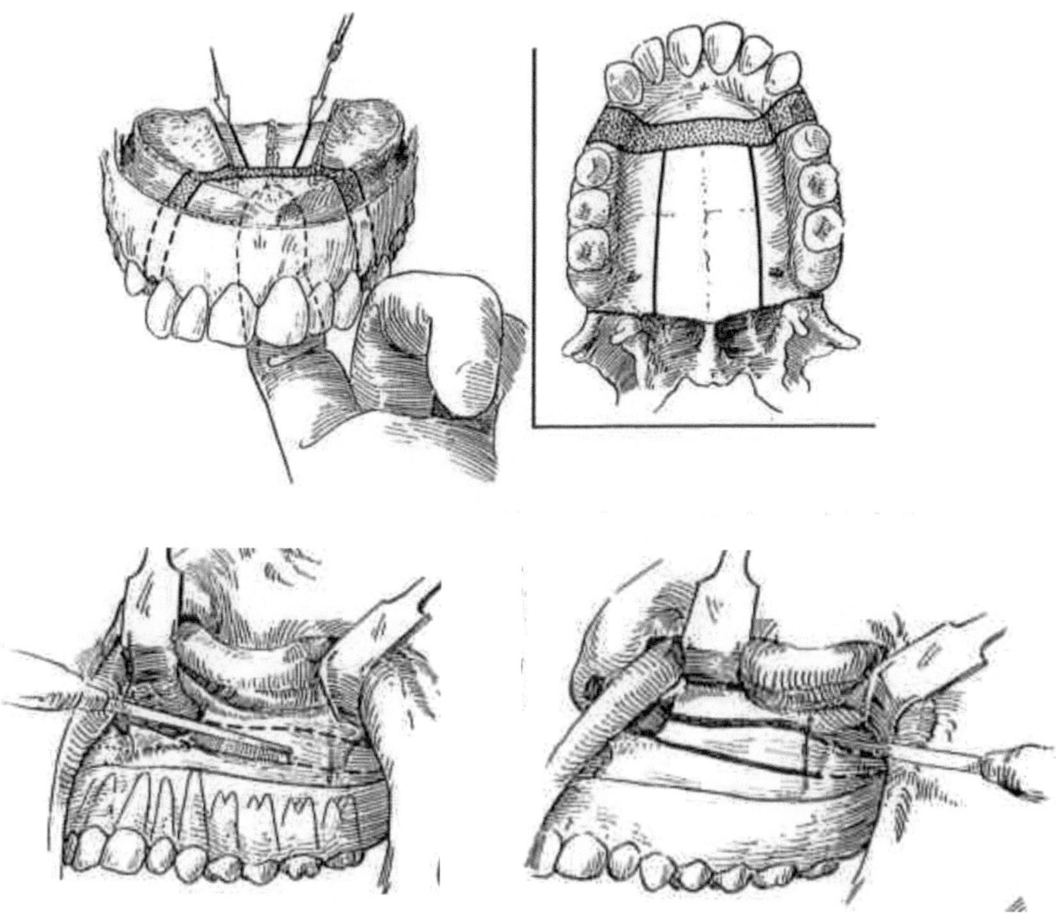

**Fig. 19.6** Le Fort I osteotomy modifications to address specific transverse or vertical discrepancies in conjunction with correction of anterior–posterior abnormalities

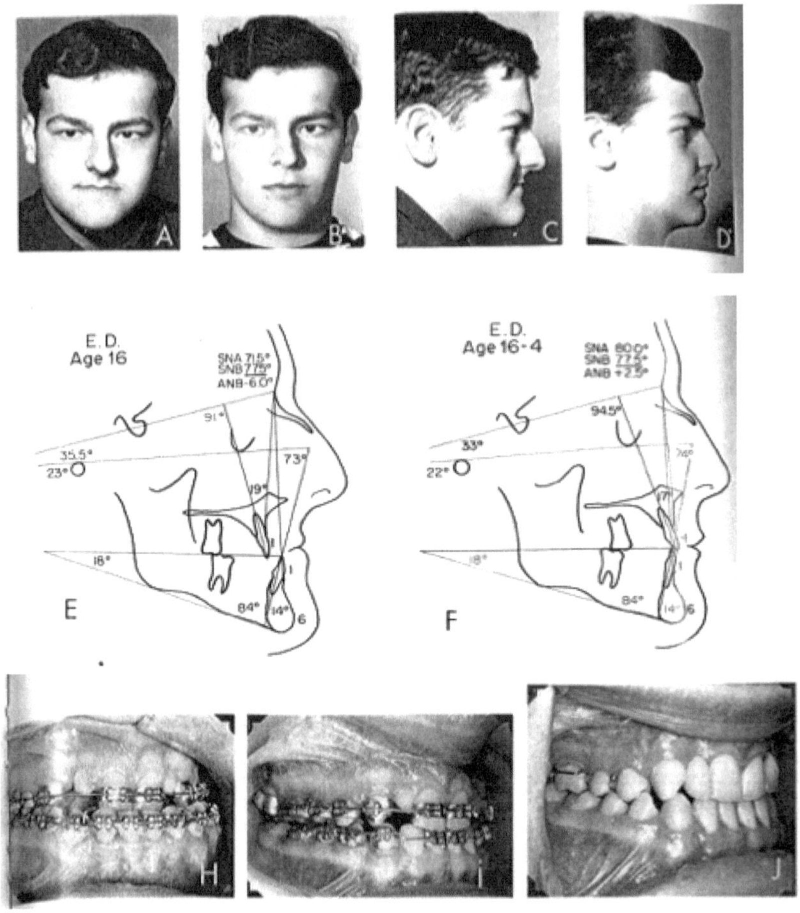


**Fig. 19.7** Le Fort I osteotomy advancement: clinical case from Dr. Bell with preoperative and postoperative facial photos, cephalometric tracings, and occlusal photos

- "In patients who display an excessive amount of gingiva and teeth in a position of repose or smiling … the maxilla can be repositioned superiorly to improve the upper lip line-to-incisor relationship. The consequent autorotation of the mandible is an effective means of increasing chin prominence."
- "Submucosal resection of the cartilaginous septum or turbinectomy, or both, may be necessary when the maxilla is superiorly repositioned in excess of 10 mm."
- Assessing the nasal cartilaginous septum at the conclusion of the procedure to ensure no buckling is present and septum remains midline. Informing the patient of increase in alar base width following maxillary advancement, and possibility for the need of future rhinoplasty.

At the conclusion of his paper, Bell acknowledges that he has just scratched the surface of the applications of this technique. He also comments that what would become orthognathic surgery is a "fertile meeting place for orthodontists and oral surgeons." Consequently, this paper laid the foundation for the basic clinical and biological principles of orthognathic surgery. Bell would later publish the first inclusive textbook for treatment of dentofacial deformities in conjunction with orthodontist William Proffit (Fig. 19.8).

This textbook not only served as the first "Bible" of orthognathic surgical techniques but also emphasized the importance of orthodontic treatment in conjunction with corrective jaw surgery.

Dr. William H. Bell was born and raised in St. Louis, Missouri. Prior to entering dental school, he served in the Navy during World War II and then graduated from St. Louis University School of Dentistry in 1954. He then underwent training in oral and maxillofacial surgery in Houston under Dr. Edward C. Hinds, who at the time was at the forefront in mandibular reconstructive surgery. He graduated in 1956 and became the first teaching fellow in oral surgery at MD Anderson Hospital in Houston. He remained as staff at the University of Texas Dental Branch/School of Dentistry until 1972. During that time, he performed many of his animal studies regarding orthognathic osteotomies to evaluate wound healing and revascularization. He was then recruited to University of Texas Southwestern in Dallas in 1972 under the supervision of Dr. Robert V. Walker. He continued his research in maxillary and mandibular osteotomies but also became well known for his research on distraction osteogenesis. Bell spent 20 years at UT Southwestern as a faculty and researcher and developed a renowned clinical orthognathic practice that incorporated weekly "dentofacial deformity" conferences that included both oral and maxillofacial surgery residents and orthodontic residents. He then transitioned in 1992 to Baylor College of Dentistry at Baylor University Medical Center and spent his final 10 years as a professor, retiring in 2002. He passed away on June 1, 2016, in Stowe, Vermont.

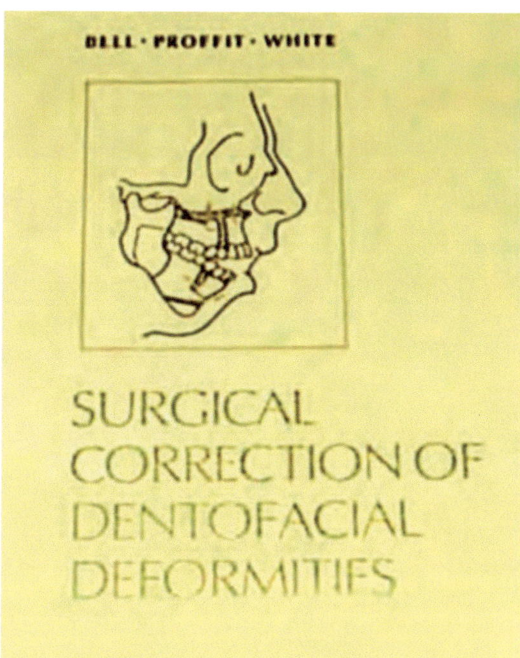


**Fig. 19.8** The first inclusive textbook that described orthognathic surgical principles and the biological basis of maxillary and mandibular osteotomies

Over the course of his career, Dr. Bell published 170 journal articles, 8 textbooks, and countless book chapters to further the study of orthognathic surgery and correction of dentofacial deformities. Many of his techniques and clinical concepts that he developed are still a part of resident training programs to this day. Bell taught and mentored hundreds of students, residents, research fellows and was truly a pioneer in the field of orthognathic surgery and within the specialty of oral and maxillofacial surgery.

## Further Reading

Bell WH. Revascularization and bone healing after anterior maxillary osteotomy. J Oral Surg. 1969;27:249.

Bell WH. Le Forte I osteotomy for correction of maxillofacial deformities. J Oral Surg. 1975;33:412–26.

Bell WH, Levy BM. Revascularization and bone healing after posterior maxillary osteotomy. J Oral Surg. 1971;29:313–20.

Bell WH, et al. Bone healing and revascularization after total maxillary osteotomy. J Oral Surg. 1975;33:253.

Kademani D, et al. Atlas of oral & maxillofacial surgery. 1st ed. St. Louis: Elsevier; 2016. p. 415–797.

Patterson R. The Le Fort fractures: René Le Fort and his work in anatomical pathology. Can J Surg. 1991;34(2):183–4.

Posnick JC. Orthognathic surgery: principles & practice. 2nd ed. Philadelphia: Elsevier; 2022. p. 33–45.

Schendel SA. Foundations: a reflection on the life of William H. Bell. Oral Surg Oral Med. 2016;122(4):375.

Wolford LA. The history of oral and maxillofacial surgery at Baylor University Medical Center. Proc (Bayl Univ Med Cent). 2004;17(1):35–41.

# Classification and Management of Mandibular Asymmetry: A Review of Past and Current Concepts

20

Emeric R. D. Boudreaux, Terry D. Taylor, and Mark E. Wong

**Abstract**

This paper analyzes the historical paper, entitled "Classification and Management of Mandibular Asymmetry," written by Hinds, Reid, and Burch. This retrospective case series follows 17 patients with mandibular asymmetry from both the University of Texas Dental Branch in Houston and Lackland Air Force Base in San Antonio, which included historical classification and accepted treatment modalities from that time. Current therapies in classification and management of mandibular asymmetry are included. In addition, special focus is made toward the original three authors, Hinds, Reid, and Burch, and their achievements in the field of orthognathic surgery. First-hand accounts of training/practice with these individuals are detailed by authors Wong and Taylor.

E. R. D. Boudreaux
East Jefferson General Hospital,
New Orleans, LA, USA

T. D. Taylor
Houston Methodist Hospital, Houston, TX, USA
e-mail: drtaylor@terrytaylor.net

M. E. Wong (✉)
Katz Department of Oral and Maxillofacial Surgery,
University of Texas Health Science Center,
Houston, TX, USA
e-mail: Mark.E.Wong@uth.tmc.edu

**Keywords**

Mandibular asymmetry · Mandibular hyperplasia · Mandibular prognathism · Edward Hinds · Loy Reid · Richard Burch

## Review of a Historical Manuscript

The paper under review is titled "Classification and Management of Mandibular Asymmetry" by Edward C. Hinds, Loy C. Reid, and Richard F. Burch. It was published in Volume 100 of the *American Journal of Surgery* in December 1960 and contained a retrospective review of a case series describing the classification and management of mandibular asymmetry. In addition to discussing the original paper, we will provide some background on the authors as pioneers in the field of orthognathic surgery and their experiences in the early days of the specialty.

This paper analyzes a total of 17 cases with mandibular asymmetry. The patients were categorized based on age of onset/age of presentation, presenting symptoms, radiographic and dental findings and associated skeletal changes such as downgrowth of the maxilla. Additional assessments were performed on the histology of the condylar head when excised, presumed etiology for asymmetry and different methods of treatment. The authors also suggested treatment outcomes as corroborative evidence for presumed causes of mandibular asymmetry.


S. R. Aziz, M. D. Turner (eds.), *Classic Papers and Pioneers in Maxillofacial and Oral Surgery*,
https://doi.org/10.1007/978-3-031-63246-4_20

Mandibular asymmetry is presented as a relatively new diagnosis without definitive criteria, since "mandibular asymmetry" as a condition had not been truly defined until 1951 by Gottlieb [1]. He described two causes of asymmetry: neoplasia involving the mandibular condyle (e.g., osteoma or osteochondroma) or "deviation prognathism," a developmental process resulting from mandibular ramus or body overgrowth. This skeletal abnormality was far less common than mandibular prognathism and warranted further study. Other possible causes of asymmetry included disturbances of growth of the condyle involving hyperplastic or prolonged growth of condylar tissue. Hinds, Reid, and Burch hoped to contribute to the literature on this condition by characterizing the radiographic and dental occlusal findings in 17 patients who presented to the University of Texas Dental Branch in Houston and Lackland Air Force Base in San Antonio. They also proceeded to describe the results of 10 out of 17 patients who underwent surgery suggesting that response to treatment would further clarify the etiology of mandibular asymmetry. Accepted therapies of that time for asymmetry included condylectomy, ramus osteotomies, body ostectomy, and local excision of the mental protuberance. However, in the series of patients treated in this series, only condylectomy, high condylar "shave," or ramus osteotomies were used to manage the asymmetry. The authors divided the causes of mandibular asymmetry into genetic or acquired conditions. They proposed the following classification in their original article:

1. Inherent (genetic)
   a. Deviation prognathism
   b. Condylar recession or absence (hypoplasia)
2. Acquired
   a. Developmental
      i. Asymmetric hyperplasia
      ii. Asymmetric hypoplasia
         1. Infection
         2. Trauma
   b. Mechanical
      i. Tumor, e.g., osteochondroma
      ii. Trauma (unilateral recession)
      iii. Surgery (unilateral recession)

Of the 17 patients, a significant number, 13, presented for examination after the age of 20 with 4 patients presenting in the fourth decade of life. Since a minority (7/17) experienced some form of malocclusion (lateral or anterior open bite, tilting of the occlusal plane), this suggested a slowly developing condition perhaps mitigated by dental compensations. Radiographic evidence of abnormality was more significant. The condyle on the affected side was "markedly enlarged" in 13/17 patients and there was evidence of morphological "distortion" in 3/17 cases. These condylar changes lead to TMJ-related problems including pain, joint noises, chewing, and range of motion compromise and ear symptoms in 12/17 patients. In 7/17 patients, clinical and radiographic evidence of significant "downgrowth" of the mandible was also evident. Despite the strong radiographic evidence of condylar hyperplasia, morphological changes to the mandibular ramus and body prompted the authors to consider alternative treatment methods.

In the late 1950s, the accepted treatment for mandibular asymmetry was a condylectomy. 3/17 patients in their series were treated in this fashion and in two patients, excessive bone and cartilage formation suggested the presence of an osteochondroma. In the last patient, the histology was reported as hyperplasia. This paper describes the role of unilateral and bilateral subcondylar osteotomies as a successful alternative to condylectomy, with the belief that once condylar changes stabilized, the resultant mandibular asymmetry could be successfully treated by addressing the mandibular deformity. This approach can be viewed as a turning point in the management of mandibular asymmetry and represents the most important point made by this publication. It suggests that the deformity is not just the result of condylar growth but additional growth of the mandibular ramus or body contributed to asymmetry. Several additional conclusions were made and are listed below:

1. Mandibular asymmetry involving condylar overgrowth can be described as either: unilateral condylar hyperplasia or deviation

prognathism (condyles being approximately the same size).
2. 15 cases were deemed unilateral condylar hyperplasia, 2 deviation prognathism.
3. Condylar hyperplasia seen in this study is most likely true hyperplasia, and not an osteoma nor osteochondroma.
4. A rare source of mandibular asymmetry can be seen with hyperplasia or hypertrophy of the ramus or body of the mandible and not localized to the condyle itself.
5. The majority of cases occur during the patient's growth period.
6. Unilateral mandibular hyperplasia is not associated with familial incidence—is acquired, not genetic in origin.
7. Earlier age of onset = more diffuse distortion, onset after maturity displays more distortion at site, in this case condylar head.
8. Mandibular asymmetry, unlike mandibular prognathism, produces many symptoms, including pain, joint noises and interference with motion.
9. Mandibular asymmetry may be treated surgically by condylectomy, subcondylar osteotomy, ostectomy in the body of the mandible, or by more complicated procedures in isolated cases. A few are benefited by prosthetic appliances and a rather significant number do not require or desire treatment.
10. Malignant disease must always remain in the differential diagnosis.

## Limitations of Study

Several weaknesses of this study include a small study population, lack of histological evaluation in all patients with radiographically enlarged condyles, and the absence of tests for determining continued growth activity, despite the availability of modalities such as serial cephalometric examinations at that time. A lack of intra-cohort controls comparing treatment outcomes following condylectomy and subcondylar osteotomies also affects the strength of the conclusions reached. In patients with TMJ symptoms, no post-operative TMJ evaluation was discussed reporting the persistence or resolution of complaints following surgery.

## Current Approach to Mandibular Asymmetry

Since the publication of this original paper in 1960, significant advancements have been made in the diagnosis, classification, and management of mandibular asymmetry. A proper history, focusing on time of presentation, associated traumatic events, and progression of growth disturbances offer valuable information. The physical examination documents location and characteristics of asymmetry with attention to facial elongation/widening/projection, maxillary cant, occlusal discrepancies, facial and dental midline alignment, additional facial asymmetries, and a comprehensive temporomandibular joint examination. Diagnostic imaging can include a preliminary panoramic radiograph, but current treatment standards utilize a cone-beam or helical computed tomography scan as the basis. Growth activity and skeletal maturation should be evaluated with single-photon emission tomography (SPECT). Advances in growth mapping are now far more sensitive and specific for identifying continued metabolic activity of the mandible with single-photon emission tomography (SPECT) having a sensitivity of 93% and specificity of 96% [2]. After surgical intervention, histological evaluation of tissue removed can be used to confirm an etiological process.

The current approach to the diagnosis and management of facial asymmetry is based on consideration of the following three causes of mandibular asymmetry: congenital, developmental, and acquired etiologies. This classification at the outset can guide diagnostic and treatment as depicted in our following chart [3] Mandibular asymmetry management: (Fig. 20.1).

Congenital asymmetries include orofacial clefts, hemifacial microsomia, neurofibromato-

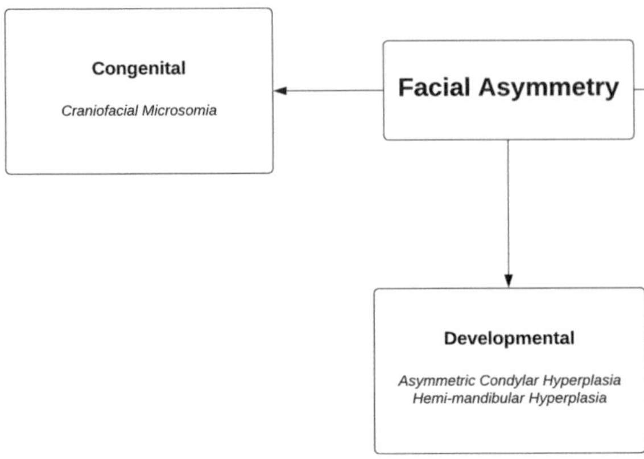


**Fig. 20.1** A simplified depiction of the main sources of mandibular (facial) asymmetry: congenital, developmental, and acquired. Congenital sources can be attributed mainly to craniofacial microsomia; developmental sources attributed to asymmetric condylar hyperplasia and hemi-mandibular hyperplasia; acquired sources are for the most part (simplified for this discussion) sequela of trauma, condylar degeneration, or neoplastic behavior

sis, congenital muscular torticollis, and unilateral coronal craniosynostosis; however, the principal cause of mandibular asymmetry is hemifacial microsomia [4]. Developmental causes resulting in asymmetry include asymmetric condylar hyperplasia and hemi-mandibular hyperplasia. These can be further subdivided into hyperplasia of the condyle, ramus, and body specifically. Acquired causes of asymmetry are found in the setting of either trauma or pathology. Trauma can produce post-traumatic condylar growth deficiencies or degenerative changes from an inflammatory mediated process. Pathological causes of mandibular asymmetry include benign condylar lesions including osteochondroma, osteoma, or lymphatic malformations of the skull base or maxillofacial regions. The surgical management for these disparate causes utilized today includes procedures to address abnormalities of the condyle requiring removal of the joint or in agreement with the concept of skeletal correction of mandibular asymmetry proposed by the original Hinds, Reid, and Burch paper, surgery of the mandibular body, ramus, and genial protuberance. The list of procedures includes condylectomy, costochondral grafting, alloplastic total joint reconstruction, distraction osteogenic lengthening of the ramus, orthognathic surgery of the ramus or mandibular body, recontouring osteoplasty of the mandible, and genioplasty (Fig. 20.2). Virtual surgical planning helps determine the position of osteotomies and size of ostectomies to achieve both skeletal and occlusal harmony, and the availability of surgical guides and patient-specific implants can facilitate the positioning and fixation of the mandible and maxilla after surgery. In our current context, the clear majority of cases with mandibular asymmetry treated by the authors of this review paper are managed with bilateral sagittal split osteotomies (BSSO) or intra-oral vertical ramus osteotomies (IVRO). Removal of the condyle followed by total joint reconstruction comprises only a handful of patients during a 40+ year professional career.

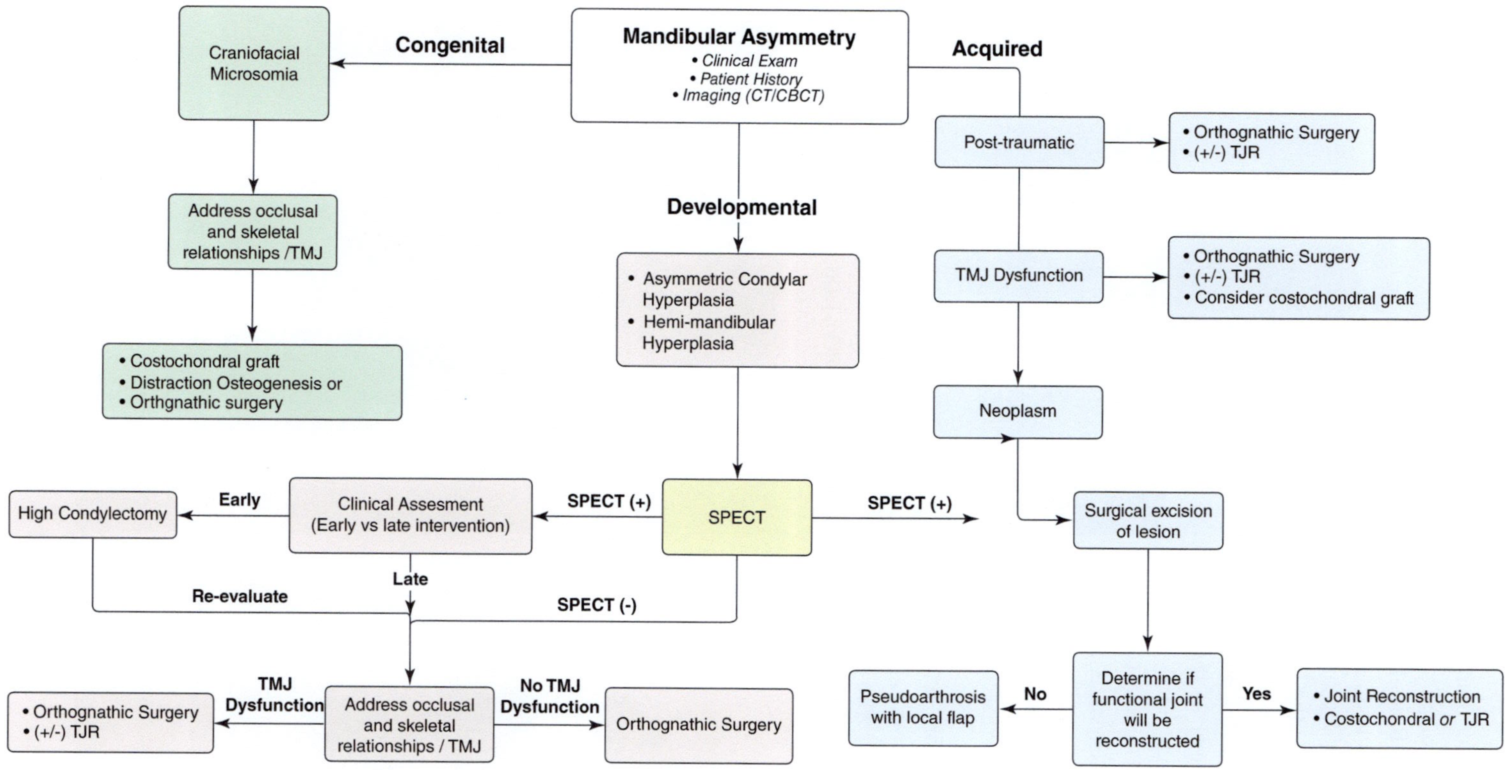


**Fig. 20.2** Flowchart depicting the algorithm for management of facial asymmetry. All initial management consists of clinical exam, patient history, and imaging (CBCT). (Green) Congenital manifestation, craniofacial microsomia, can be treated with costochondral graft (TMJ) and distraction osteogenesis or sometimes with orthognathic surgery (BSSO or IVRO, ±maxillary osteotomy). (Red) Developmental sources (hyperplasia) can be further evaluated with SPECT. If SPECT displays growth, the decision to perform early intervention (high condylectomy) can be made. Following early intervention or if SPECT displays resolution of growth, evaluation of occlusal, skeletal, and TMJ is performed. From this point, if no TMJ dysfunction is present, patient can be treated with orthognathic surgery alone. If TMJ dysfunction is present, the case can be made to treat the patient with orthognathic surgery. (Blue) Acquired sources can be attributed to 3 causes (for this discussion). Post-traumatic asymmetry can be treated with orthognathic surgery ± TJR. TMJ dysfunction leading to degeneration of the condylar head and mandibular asymmetry can be treated with orthognathic surgery with or without TJR—in these cases, costochondral graft should be considered. Neoplastic processes, which will also result in SPECT as metabolic activity, are initially treated with surgical excision of lesion. Following removal of the condylar head, a decision should be made whether to reconstruct the anatomical space with either soft tissue alone—resulting in a pseudoarthrosis or with a total joint reconstructio using either a costochondral graft or alloplastic joint reconstruction system. *CT* computed tomography, *CBCT* cone-beam computed tomography, *SPECT* single-photon emission computed tomography, *TMJ* temporomandibular joint, *TJR* total joint reconstruction (alloplastic joint)

## The Authors of the Historical Paper

The three authors of this paper published in 1960 in the *American Journal of Surgery* were Edward Hinds, DDS, MD, Loy Reid, DDS, and Richard Burch, DDS. Dr. Hinds (Fig. 20.3) was Professor and Chairman of the Department of Oral and Maxillofacial Surgery at the University of Texas Dental Branch in Houston, Dr. Reid (Fig. 20.4) was a second-year resident, and Dr. Burch (Fig. 20.5) was a Colonel in the USAF Dental Corps and Chief of the Oral Surgery Service at Lackland Military Training Center in San Antonio, Texas. He also served as the Oral Surgery Consultant to the USAF 6110th Hospital Group and was an occasional visitor to the Houston program to teach residents and perform surgery.

Edward Copas Hinds was born on May 10, 1917, in Park Rapids, Minnesota. His father, Frederick W. Hinds was a dentist who graduated from the University of Minnesota. In 1926, Dr. Frederick Hinds decided to leave private practice

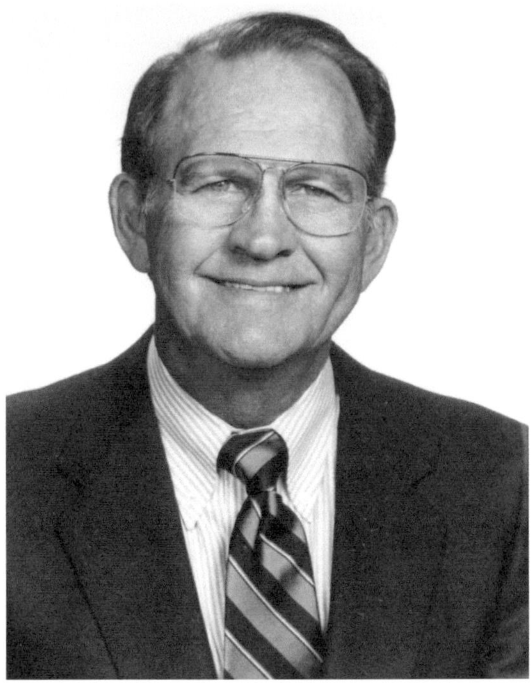

**Fig. 20.4** Loy C. Reid, DDS, MS

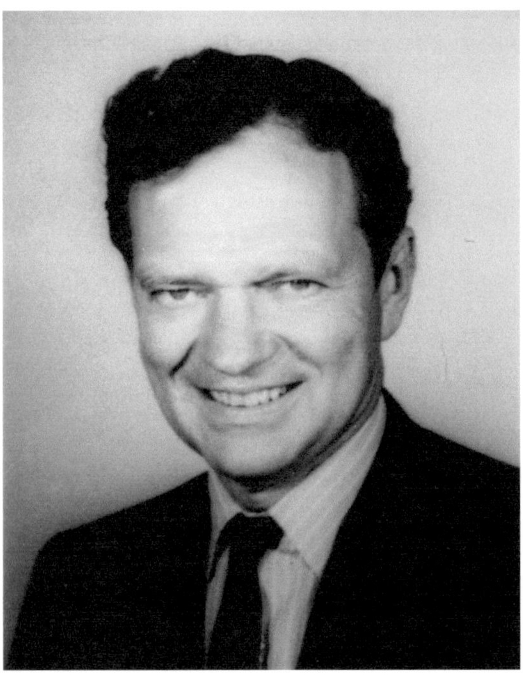

**Fig. 20.3** Edward C. Hinds, DDS, MD

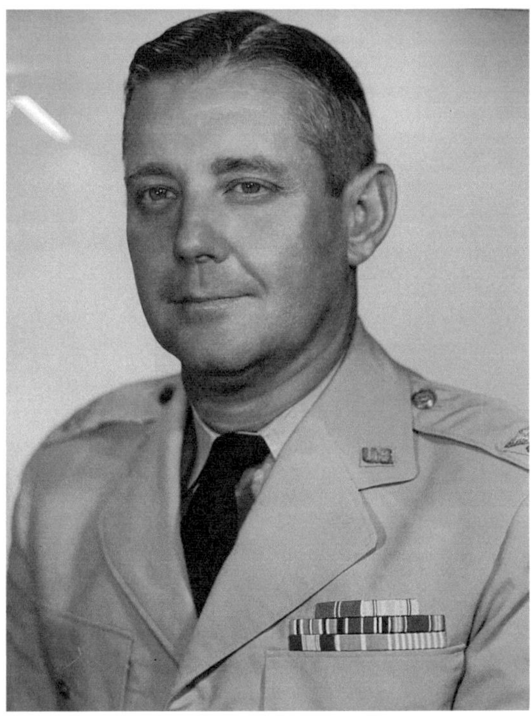

**Fig. 20.5** Richard F. Burch, DDS

and join academia at the Baylor University College of Dentistry where he became Dean in 1927 and remained in that position until 1943. Edward Hinds grew up in Dallas and attended college at Baylor University in Waco, Texas, before returning to dental school at Baylor. He excelled scholastically and graduated in 1940 with his DDS, before deciding to pursue a medical degree. He was admitted to Baylor College of Medicine which was originally in Waco but relocated to Houston in 1943 when the MD Anderson Foundation invited the medical school to join the newly formed Texas Medical Center as a cornerstone institution. The College of Medicine opened in Houston July 12, 1943, in a converted Sears, Roebuck and Co. building, with 131 students, including Dr. Edward Hinds. Upon graduation from medical school in 1945, Dr. Hinds completed an internship at Parkland Hospital in Dallas before enlisting in the US Navy Medical Corps. In 1948, Michael E. DeBakey, M.D., the renowned cardiothoracic surgeon, joined the faculty as chair of the Department of Surgery, and Dr. Hinds was accepted to a general surgery residency under Dr. DeBakey from 1948 to 1953. In his final year of residency, he was appointed as Department Chair of Oral Surgery in 1952 at the University of Texas School of Dentistry, later renamed as the University of Texas Dental Branch in 1955. Dr. Hinds was board certified by the American Board of Oral Surgery in 1952 and the American Board of Surgery in 1956. In addition to chairing the department and developing an undergraduate curriculum for dental students, Dr. Hinds started an oral surgery residency in 1949 while still a general surgery resident. Obviously, the first oral surgery residents were expected to have some degree of competence and the ability to operate independently. Drs. Joseph Kuebel and Bruno Kwapis were already in training at Charity Hospital in New Orleans and Indiana University Medical Center, respectively, and agreed to rotate to Houston to help start the training program. Dr. Hinds served as Program Director from 1949 to 1965 before relinquishing the role to Dr. John Pleasants, a retired army oral surgeon. Without the formal training of an oral (and maxillofacial) surgeon, Dr. Hinds focused his expertise and attention on head and neck pathology and in the developing field of correction of dentofacial deformities. The ramus osteotomy to manage mandibular prognathism was a "favorite" operation before research into the viability of maxillary osteotomies was performed by Dr. William Bell. Dr. Bell completed the Houston oral surgery program in 1957 and joined the faculty upon completion of his training to continue his research which contributed to the foundation of orthognathic surgery. Dr. Hinds cemented his legacy as one of the pioneers in orthognathic surgery when he and another resident protégé, Dr. John Kent, published their seminal textbook *Surgical Treatment of Developmental Jaw Deformities* in 1972. Dr. Hinds continued as Department Chair until 1983, navigating the increasing complex environment of the Texas Medical Center as it grew into the largest medical center in the world with competing interests from two medical schools and a host of hospitals. In 1989 after a few years of declining health, Edward C. Hinds passed away from a heart attack at Methodist Hospital, leaving his wife Dorothy and three children including the noted cartoonist Bill Hinds, creator of the syndicated comic strip "Tank McNamara" and "Buzzy Beamer."

Loy Campbell Reid was a Texas native who was born on January 16, 1928, in Nacogdoches, Texas, a town approximately 140 miles northeast of Houston. He attended Steven F. Austin State University for undergraduate studies and the University of Texas Dental Branch graduating in 1955. He practiced general dentistry for 3 years in Austin, before being accepted to the oral surgery residency in Houston in 1958. Dr. Reid completed the program in 1961 and was board certified by the American Board of Oral Surgery the following year. His personnel file which we were able to recover in our department archives documents his communications with Dr. Hinds expressing his interest and willingness to accept a $100 per month stipend and $120 per month housing and food allowance. Of significant interest, especially by comparison to today's standards, is that he was married with four dependents when he started his program. Upon completion of his residency, he entered private practice in Corpus Christi, Texas. His early years in practice reflected some of the challenges oral surgeons without medical degrees faced against competing interests from other medical specialties. Letters between him and Dr. Hinds describe problems with credentialing for hospital procedures and the advice provided by Dr. Hinds. Dr. Reid practiced until 1994 before retiring. He passed away at the age of 79 in 2007.

Dr. Burch was a native of Oklahoma. He was born and raised in small towns, first Quinton and later Stilwell, OK. He was the first Air Force surgeon to become a diplomat of the American Board of Oral Surgery and later served on the Examination Committee. While on active duty in the USAF, he was responsible for starting the very first oral surgery training program at Lackland Air Force Base and served as its Chief from 1953 to 1960. He and Dr. Hinds met when Dr. Hinds was appointed as the Consultant to the Surgeon General of the US Air Force. Dr. Burch was known to come to Houston to give lectures and participate in surgery. Dr. Robert Johnson was one of the first oral surgery residents under Dr. Burch and when contacted for this historical review article, he had the following comments about him. "Colonel Burch was a unique no nonsense man with a straight forward way. In 1957 I was working for him and we moved to Wilford Hall. He encouraged me to consider OMS and even had me join Toastmasters to learn and feel comfortable with lecturing. He was tough and pretty inflexible but dedicated to establishing a good residency. Which he did." A review of Dr. Burch's publications reflects broad interests in a variety of conditions, but notably, he published a case report on intra-oral one stage osteotomy for the correction of mandibular prognathism and a description of unilateral condylar hyperplasia and hypoplasia of the contralateral mandibular body in 1960. This was the same time he co-authored the article which is the subject of this review. Following retirement from the military, Dr. Burch moved to Arizona where he practiced briefly in Tucson, but shortly after joined the University of Kentucky faculty where he taught until 1975. Dr. Burch passed away at the age of 69 in 1977 and is interred at Arlington National Cemetery.

## Special Perspective from Dr. Terry Taylor

Dr. Taylor, one of the pre-eminent orthognathic surgeons of our times and a co-author of this paper, was a resident under Dr. Hinds. He offers the following personal account of his experience with Dr. Hinds.

> Ed Hinds was not a talkative or flamboyant person, at least in our presence. My earliest interaction with him was looking over his shoulder in the central area of the Oral Surgery office suite at the Dental Branch (circa 1978) as he put together projection slides (Kodachromes) for a presentation. I was very interested and wanting to know more, I blurted out a question, "Is that preop or postop"? Without looking up and in a neutral tone of voice, he simply replied, "I once fired a secretary for asking that question."
>
> He was pretty "hands off" when it came to working up cases, assuming the upper level resident on his service was up to the challenge. It wasn't uncommon to be handed the x-rays and models less than 24 hours before the case was scheduled to begin. Lab work, splint construction (and admitting the patient to Methodist that evening) would then be accomplished before the OR time the following morning.
>
> While he was an accomplished orthognathic surgeon, "his" (VRO) operation was the clear favorite. He would allow the resident to do one side of pretty much every case. We would do the bilateral subcondylar osteotomies, via the "Hinds (retromandibular) approach", usually within 45 minutes to one hour. A "sagging condyle" on a postop x-ray, while uncommon, was never a concern to him. His last OR case, to my knowledge, was one that I invited him to do with myself and Theeralaksna Suddhasthira, DDS, PhD. (She wanted to return to Thailand, having done a case with Dr. Hinds.)
>
> Mary Francis Jones was "his" nurse at Methodist. If you respected Dr. Hinds, she was your best friend. If she thought you were at all disrespectful ... well, best not to go there.
>
> While I do not use the subcondylar or vertical ramus osteotomies very much in my current practice, many of the basic surgical techniques in terms

of instrumentation and soft tissue management, I learned from him and use every time I am in the OR.

The only time I saw him appear sad was when he understood he was retiring as Department Chairman at the Dental Branch.

## References

1. Hinds EC, Reid LC, Burch RJ. Classification and management of mandibular asymmetry. Am J Surg. 1960;100:825–34. https://doi.org/10.1016/0002-9610(60)90513-4.
2. López BDF, Corral SCM. Comparison of planar bone scintigraphy and single photon emission computed tomography for diagnosis of active condylar hyperplasia. J Craniomaxillofac Surg. 2016;44(1):70–4. https://doi.org/10.1016/j.jcms.2015.10.026.
3. Veeranki S, Park JH, Pruzansky D, Takagi M, Tai K. A current review of asymmetry. J Clin Orthod. 2018;52(6–7):325–41.
4. Srivastava D, Singh H, Mishra S, Sharma P, Kapoor P, Chandra L. Facial asymmetry revisited: part I—diagnosis and treatment planning. J Oral Biol Craniofac Res. 2018;8(1):7–14. https://doi.org/10.1016/j.jobcr.2017.04.010.

# Index





S. R. Aziz, M. D. Turner (eds.), *Classic Papers and Pioneers in Maxillofacial and Oral Surgery*,
https://doi.org/10.1007/978-3-031-63246-4

**W**

MIX
Papier aus verantwortungsvollen Quellen
Paper from responsible sources
FSC® C105338

If you have any concerns about our products,
you can contact us on
**ProductSafety@springernature.com**

In case Publisher is established outside the EU,
the EU authorized representative is:
**Springer Nature Customer Service Center GmbH**
**Europaplatz 3, 69115 Heidelberg, Germany**

Printed by Libri Plureos GmbH
in Hamburg, Germany